EATING WELL
after Weight Loss Surgery

EATING WELL
after Weight Loss Surgery

Over 150 Delicious Low-Fat
High-Protein Recipes to Enjoy in the Weeks,
Months, and Years after Surgery

Patt Levine and Michele Bontempo

Consulting Nutritionist, Meredith Urban-Skuro, MS, RD, CDN

Da Capo

LIFE
LONG

Copyright © 2018 by Patricia Levine and Michele Bontempo
Cover design by Alex Camlin
Cover image © Stockfood
Cover copyright © 2018 Hachette Book Group, Inc.

Da Capo Press
Hachette Book Group
1290 Avenue of the Americas, New York, NY 10104
dacapopress.com
@DaCapoPress

Printed in the United States of America

Originally published in paperback by Marlowe & Company in July 2004

Revised Edition: December 2018

Published by Da Capo Lifelong Books, an imprint of Perseus Books, LLC, a subsidiary of Hachette Book Group, Inc. The Da Capo Lifelong Books name and logo is a trademark of the Hachette Book Group.

The publisher is not responsible for websites (or their content) that are not owned by the publisher.

Print book interior design by Amy Quinn

Library of Congress Cataloging-in-Publication Data has been applied for.

ISBNs: 978-0-7382-3504-2 (paperback), 978-0-7382-3505-9 (ebook)

LSC-C

10 9 8 7 6 5 4 3 2 1

Contents

4 Main Course 57

Chicken Entrées

Turkey Entrées

Seafood Entrées

Vegetarian Entrées

Foreword by Jon Gould, MD

Bariatric and metabolic surgery has come a long way since the early days in the 1960s. Over the past fifty years, many bariatric surgical procedures have come and gone. Some of these procedures just didn't work (such as horizontal gastroplasty, known in the 1980s as stomach stapling), and others led to an unacceptable rate of nutritional or other issues (jejunoileal bypass). Modern and minimally invasive alternatives have arrived to replace procedures that are now rarely performed (for example, vertical banded gastroplasty has been replaced by the laparoscopic adjustable gastric band and the sleeve gastrectomy). The gastric bypass is the longest-standing bariatric procedure still commonly performed to this day. In the United States, the most commonly performed bariatric surgical procedure is the sleeve gastrectomy, followed by gastric bypass, laparoscopic adjustable gastric band, and biliopancreatic diversion/duodenal, switch respectively. New endoscopic alternatives are appearing and slowly gaining popularity. These include such options as the intragastric balloon, endoscopic sleeve gastroplasty (like a sleeve gastrectomy with an endoscope), and the endoscopically placed duodenal-jejunal bypass liner. (Each of these procedures has its own advantages and disadvantages, and many factors go into recommending a particular procedure to a particular patient.) In 2014, it was estimated that nearly 200,000 bariatric surgical procedures were performed in the United States.

Bariatric surgery is safer than it has ever been. When I first started performing bariatric surgery in the late 1990s, we would quote a mortality rate of around 1 percent following bariatric surgery. In 2017, at accredited bariatric surgery centers in the United States, the mortality rate was 0.1 percent (that's a 90 percent reduction). Bariatric surgery has been shown to lead to improved health, with high rates of remission of type 2 diabetes, gastroesophageal reflux, and obstructive sleep apnea, to name just a few conditions. Patients experience an improved quality of life and sense of well-being. Bariatric surgery actually decreases a person's risk of dying over time. And, to consider the financial impact, obesity is costly (about $1 of every $10 spent on health care in the United States is related to obesity), and bariatric surgery has been demonstrated to be cost effective. All professional societies that represent physicians who manage severely obese patients (the American College of Cardiology/American Heart Association, American Association of Clinical Endocrinologists, the Obesity Society, and more) recommend bariatric surgery referral and evaluation for morbidly obese patients who are considered appropriate surgical candidates.

Despite all of the above, bariatric surgery is vastly underutilized, and less than 1 percent of eligible candidates undergo surgery each year. There are likely many reasons for this. There are misperceptions that bariatric surgery is risky or that patients gain all of their weight back. There is also a lack of understanding about the causes of obesity, and how difficult it is for patients to overcome this condition—even among health-care providers. Primary care physicians generally underemphasize obesity treatments, overestimate the risks of bariatric surgery, and have a poor understanding of the ideal surgical candidate or when to refer. Moreover, access to bariatric surgery services is poor in many parts of the country, most often related to unreasonable insurance requirements or restrictions, or a complete lack of coverage. At the same time, obesity has become more and more prevalent worldwide. It's estimated that one third of adults in the United States have obesity.

Obesity is a complex, chronic, and progressive disease resulting from multiple genetic and environmental factors. People affected by severe obesity are resistant to long-term weight loss through diet and exercise. When an obese person loses weight through dieting, his or her body will reduce energy expenditure so as to conserve calories (the body is reacting to a state of relative starvation). With dietary weight loss, the amount of dietary fat the body burns is reduced by approximately 50 percent. Because the body thinks that it is not getting enough food, the body reacts to this state of decreased energy intake by increasing appetite. During a diet, as the metabolism decreases, the ability to efficiently store fat increases, and appetite increases, weight regain is inevitable. Unfortunately, many of these changes persist long term, which can contribute to weight gain in excess of the starting point for some patients. The National Institutes of Health Experts Panel recognized that long-term weight loss is nearly impossible for those affected by severe obesity by any means other than metabolic and bariatric surgery.

Over the past seventeen years as a bariatric surgeon, I have talked to thousands of people who have struggled with obesity for much of their life. Although everyone's personal path to weight loss surgery is different, there are common themes. Prior to considering surgery, many people have successfully lost weight—sometimes a lot of weight. All of them have gained that weight back, usually despite an ongoing commitment to a diet or exercise program that seemed to work at first but at some point just stopped working. Many patients question whether it has really come to the point where they actually need to have surgery to finally overcome obesity. Many have considered surgery for years. I have heard patients wonder aloud whether surgery is the "easy way out" or if it means they are "giving up." The decision to pursue bariatric surgery is not made lightly. It is far from the "easy way out," and requires discipline and commitment to succeed. We often speak of bariatric surgery as a tool that can be used by patients and their bariatric team to help overcome the disease of obesity. Just like any other tool, it needs to be used correctly to be effective. A proper diet and approach to nutrition is one of the most important aspects of a surgical approach to obesity. Without attention to basic nutritional and dietary principles, the outcomes following bariatric surgery will be impaired.

When compared to diets, bariatric surgery is more effective at maintaining weight loss long term. This is in part because these procedures lead to metabolic and biologic changes that are different than those described for dieting alone. Weight loss following bariatric surgery does not reduce energy expenditure or the amount of calories the body burns. In fact, some bariatric procedures may even lead to an *increased* metabolic rate and energy expenditure. Following surgery, energy intake and calorie consumption is decreased through anatomic and biologic factors: Bariatric surgical procedures of the stomach decrease the capacity to eat a large meal, and in some procedures, the ingested nutrients are inefficiently absorbed. In addition, bariatric surgery leads to increased production of certain gut hormones that interact with the brain to reduce hunger and lead to a prolonged sense of fullness after eating. These bariatric surgery–induced changes in the metabolism and in the way the body responds to a meal are a critical distinction from what occurs during and following weight loss that occurs through other mechanisms. It is why these procedures are considered to be both bariatric *and* metabolic surgical procedures. The word *bariatric* is derived from the Greek word *baros*, meaning "weight." As you can see, weight loss is only part of what distinguishes bariatric surgery as the most effective tool for long-term and significant weight loss. The metabolic component is very important.

The fact that bariatric surgical procedures can lead to sustained weight loss over a very long period of time (decades) has been established. What is underappreciated is the effort and commitment that patients need to achieve these durable weight-loss outcomes. I am of the opinion that the toughest time for patients is from about one to three years post-op. This is the time when the weight loss has tapered, you don't have as frequent visits with your bariatric team, and many foods that you may have poorly tolerated at first are becoming easier for you to consume. Limited or unappealing food options make it hard for patients to adhere to the recommended diet, which is high in protein and low in fat. Bariatric surgery programs are great at educating patients as to how much protein they need, what vitamins they should take, and how much water they should drink. What we don't do as well is help patients understand and learn how to eat a bariatric appropriate diet, and still eat real food that tastes good. I have read Patt and Michelle's cookbook with great interest. The nutritional advice is spot on. The recipes are unique and sound fantastic. I tried the Omelet à la Quebec. I'm not much of a cook, but this one was easy, and it was really good! I hope you enjoy reading the advice in this book and the recipes that follow as much as I have. Patt's tips and insight into things she experienced and what she did to overcome these issues is helpful advice. Remember, bariatric surgery is just a tool. If used appropriately every day, it can be the key to helping you overcome obesity and changing your life for good.

Jon Gould, MD, is Professor of Surgery and the Alonzo P. Walker Chair in General Surgery at the Medical College of Wisconsin. He has a national reputation as a bariatric surgeon and minimally invasive foregut surgeon.

Introduction

THE WEIGHT WARS

I WAS NOT ALWAYS fat. In fact, I was a skinny kid. In my teens and early twenties, I loved my curves. But once I started working, I started gaining—a couple of pounds here, a couple of pounds there. So, I tried diet pills. They worked for a while, but I was so manic and moody while taking them, no one could stand me. When I went off them, I gained all my weight back, plus some. Then I tried dieting. You know, grapefruit, broiled steak, and salad, and I never, never ate more than the guys I was dating (one of the golden oldie definitions of "being a lady"). Then I met my husband, a great guy with a great appetite. Any amount that I ate was less than he could put away. So, I started gaining and gaining and gaining. I tried Weight Watchers, lost 40 pounds, hit a plateau, and gained it all back and more. I tried going to the gym. That certainly helped, but once my career started taking off and I was working nights, and weekends, and traveling constantly, exercise became erratic, then nonexistent. So, I gained. Then I tried the Atkins diet, which was perfect for me because I'm a real carnivore. The first time I tried it, I tested purple all the time (that means that I successfully put myself into ketosis, which is the goal), but I barely lost anything. Then I gained. I tried Atkins again. This time I lost 40 pounds, hit a plateau, and gained it all back plus some. Sound familiar?

Over a period of about twenty years, I had more than doubled my weight. I weighed over 345 pounds. I could barely walk a block without stopping to rest. I couldn't fit in theater or airplane seats. I actually broke furniture. After a bout with pneumonia, which landed me in the hospital for over a week, my primary care physician suggested that I consider weight-reduction surgery. My pulmonologist concurred. So, I did research, talked to a number of people who had undergone the surgery, and decided to do it.

My doctor referred me to Dr. William Inabnet, a renowned expert in bariatric surgery and a thoroughly professional and truly compassionate man. He and his staff seemed to understand exactly what I was going through and how I had gotten to this point, without being judgmental. We decided that I was a good candidate for laparoscopic Lap-Band bariatric surgery. The surgery was successful, but then the real battle began. As Dr. Inabnet and his staff reminded me, the surgery is only a tool. Now I had to rethink not only the amount that I ate, but the kinds of foods that I ate and, oh, yeah, start exercising.

Cooking has always been one of my greatest passions—I think I started cooking when I was eight years old. And once I discovered that cooking for other people brought me unconditional approval, well, let's just say that it became a defining part of my persona. Whereas cooking had once played a major role in my weight gain, now I was determined that it would be a significant factor in my weight loss. You see,

I love a challenge in the kitchen. For years, I had whipped up gourmet dishes around other people's likes and dislikes, allergies and restrictions. Now, I would put that talent to work for me.

I developed a high-protein, low-fat eating plan with virtually no "bad" carbohydrates. I allowed myself only "good" carbs from fruit and vegetables. The hard part was dealing with the restrictions for the first four months after surgery (but more about that later). Did it work? The answer is yes, although it's still a work in progress. I have lost a significant amount of weight, and I'm looking and feeling pretty terrific, if I do say so myself. I've even started wearing clothes that I haven't been able to get into for years. And what's amazing is that, because of my ongoing weight-loss adventure, I wrote this cookbook to help other people on their road to weight loss in the weeks, months, and years after surgery. To my great pleasure, it's become a go-to resource for other patients and health professionals. Now, I've updated my book to reflect the latest recommendations for bariatric surgery patients and share brand-new recipes I hope you and your whole family will love.

DEPRIVE MYSELF? NOT ME

Let's face it, one of the reasons most people become candidates for bariatric surgery is that we love to eat. As a self-described "foodie," I admit that I was worried when my nutritionist, Meredith Urban-Skuro, told me about the very restrictive way I would have to eat in the first months after surgery—low-fat food, pureed to the consistency of mush or chopped up in tiny bits. The suggested menus she showed me looked like a hospital soft diet—totally tasteless mush. When I was being kind, I referred to it as baby food. When I was being cynical, I called it sludge.

But just because a food's texture is bland, that doesn't mean its taste has to be. So, I set out to see if I could cook low-fat dishes tasty enough to stand up to pureeing or mincing, recipes that not only pleased, but also excited, my palate. As an added complication, I needed to cook for my husband at the same time.

My best friend, Michele, curious about the post-op restrictions on my diet, asked to taste some of the recipes I had developed. She immediately challenged me to write a cookbook for other bariatric surgery patients and offered to help.

This cookbook is proof that you can cook delicious food that not only satisfies your postsurgical guidelines, but also satisfies your taste buds. Yes, there is added work if you are cooking for others as well as yourself, but we've tried to keep it to a minimum. You can use these recipes the way they are written, or use them as a basis for experimenting to create new ones that suit your personal taste.

When I told Meredith and my surgeon that I was writing a cookbook for weight-reduction surgery patients, they were really excited.

But Meredith warned me. "Patt, I know that you are a very sophisticated cook, but not everyone who is going to use this cookbook will be, so don't make it too complicated or esoteric."

I said, "C'mon, get serious, people who aren't into cooking won't start cooking just because they had the surgery."

That's when Meredith told me something that surprised me. She found that many patients had discovered that unless they had control over what they ate, they ran into some problems; for instance, they ate too much because they couldn't control portion sizes; they didn't know how the food was prepared, so they ate unexpected fats, sugars, and other ingredients that created digestive distress. For these reasons, many of those patients *were* starting to cook seriously for the first time after surgery.

So, whether you have always been cooking or you are just starting to cook for the first time, I promise that you will enjoy using this cookbook. It will show you how to make delicious, satisfying food that will help you achieve and maintain your weight-loss goals over a long period of time.

ABOUT THIS BOOK: YOU *CAN* TURN MUSH INTO MAGIC

Let's be honest, not everything purees well. I admit it; we had a couple of real disasters while we were developing and testing these recipes. The nice thing about this cookbook is that it progresses along with your eating program—these dishes taste terrific whether they're pureed, chopped up, or served as solid food.

Our cookbook runs the gamut from breakfast and brunch dishes to soups, entrées, and vegetables. Plus, you'll find an entire section on sauces that includes both savory and sweet toppings. And speaking of sweets, we've come up with a number of sweet indulgences that are completely allowable as well as incredibly luscious.

These recipes are high in protein, contain no added sugars, are low in fat, and contain only complex carbohydrates from fruits and vegetables. Therefore, they are protein-rich, low-calorie, and have virtually no "bad carbs." What they do have is enough flavor and variety to keep you from feeling deprived. And, we didn't realize until the book was finished, all the recipes are very nearly gluten-free! If you are avoiding gluten, swap gluten-free tamari for soy sauce in the few recipes that call for it, and make sure your stock and broth choices don't contain any hidden wheat. (Do be aware that any time you modify a recipe, the nutritional information may change.)

Because this cookbook is a collaborative effort, it offers a huge amount of variety. You see, Michele and I have very different tastes in cooking and eating. She likes spicy stuff, such as curries and hot peppers. I like fruit and meat combinations and subtle seasonings. But we both agree on using high-quality ingredients. By developing these recipes together, we came up with many truly original and delectable new dishes.

We offer a wide range of recipes in each category. You'll find variations on classic French and Italian cuisine, exotic Indian and Caribbean dishes, and recipes with Asian and Mexican influences, as well as good old American comfort food. While many of our recipes are quick and uncomplicated, some require longer cooking times or specialized steps—those are the ones that I call "Sunday cooking"—you know, the foods you cook when you have more time, which taste even better reheated the second day. You'll be amazed at how we created some of the richest-tasting dishes without lots of fat or calories. Better than that, we came up with a luscious substitute for mashed potatoes that's so good even meat-and-potato guys love it.

Most of our recipes are designed to serve four people, so if you're cooking for others, they can enjoy the same foods as you're eating. Of course, you'll be eating such a small amount that there may be leftovers. (Why not puree them and reheat them for lunch the next day?)

At the bottom of each recipe you'll find preparation and serving instructions for you to follow at each post-op stage, whether you've had a Lap-Band, gastric sleeve, gastric bypass, or biliopancreatic diversion with duodenal switch (BPD-DS) procedure. In addition, you'll find portion-size suggestions to help you cook for people who aren't eating a limited diet.

Because these recipes are so delicious and interesting, we think that you and your family are going to enjoy this cookbook for years and years, even after you come to the end of your postsurgical food restrictions.

THE ROAD TO SUCCESS

Needless to say, your weight-loss journey will be unique to you, and it will depend on a number of factors. Once again, as my doctor always reminds me, the surgery is only a tool. Changing your eating and exercise habits are equally important. While we can't do anything to help you burn those calories, we can give you a new way to cook and eat. You won't feel deprived, because it's absolutely delicious. And since it doesn't restrict you to just a few limited types of food, it's easy and healthy enough to follow for a long time, even the rest of your life.

Since I had my surgery, I've experienced a steady weight loss that has made me very happy. The biggest surprise was my husband (our primary guinea pig), who did not have the surgery. By going on a modified version of this eating plan (eating these recipes for breakfast and dinner), he lost a total of 45 pounds. He's living proof that this cookbook works for *anyone* who needs to lose weight.

I am very happy that I decided to have bariatric surgery and I find that almost every day I reach a new, small goal. My life, which had become so restrictive due to my weight, is now full of new possibilities. It's wonderful to once more be able to do the things I used to take for granted when I was slimmer.

Michele and I hope that this cookbook will help you find all the success that you wish for and that you will enjoy every meal that you prepare from this cookbook along the way.

Advice from a Nutritionist

by Meredith Urban-Skuro, MS, RD, CDN

WHO SAYS IT has to be difficult to find food to eat after weight-loss surgery? It may be a little challenging in the beginning, but eventually you will be able to eat almost everything in moderation. I think that this cookbook can definitely help.

There are specific guidelines that need to be adhered to after surgery to prevent complications. Each bariatric practice may do things a little differently. Always check with your surgeon and nutritionist first, as the guidelines in this book may vary from where you had your surgery.

- For the first week, a liquid diet consisting of protein drinks and noncalorie beverages is usually recommended. In Weeks 2 and 3, a pureed, blended diet is recommended to lessen the chances of an obstruction caused by large particles of food. Obstructions can cause discomfort and may lead to vomiting. When pureeing foods, you may need to add more liquid (water, broth, or milk) in addition to the sauce to make it a better consistency. Advancing to solid foods can usually occur between four and five weeks after surgery. This book features very specific week-by-week preparation and portion-size guidelines at the bottom of each recipe, which can help you manage your diet progression. Check with your doctor or nutritionist on how to advance your diet. Although certain serving sizes are noted, don't force yourself to finish your plate if you are feeling too full.
- Chewing is key! Relax, enjoy, and taste the food that you are consuming. I encourage all my patients to chew at least *twenty-five times*. Solid food should be cut to the size of a fifth of a fingernail or smaller. If you eat too fast, don't chew your food well, or try to progress to solid food too quickly, you may overfill and vomit.
- Mealtime should take no more than thirty minutes. I recommend three meals and one to two healthy snacks during the day. Remember to measure and weigh your food so you are aware of the portion size you are eating.
- The nutritional emphasis in this cookbook is on protein foods. However, we do encourage a variety of foods and well-balanced meals. A strong emphasis needs to be placed on choosing high-protein foods. Protein is essential for growth, repair, and formation of new tissue. Protein aids in wound healing, maintains lean body mass, is a source of energy, and helps prevent protein malnutrition.
- Great protein choices are meat, fish, poultry, eggs, cheese, milk, yogurt, beans, soy, and nuts. Solid, dense, protein-rich foods allow you to feel satiated for a longer period of time.

Make sure to choose lean cuts of meat, trim off the fat, and take the skin off the poultry to reduce your fat intake.

- ➤ After weight-loss surgery, protein needs vary depending on the type of surgery you have undergone. After the Lap-Band, aim for 50 to 60 grams of protein per day. After a gastric sleeve or gastric bypass, aim for 50 to 70 grams of protein per day. After a BPD-DS, aim for 80 to 120 grams of protein a day. Not meeting your protein needs can lead to protein malnutrition—a condition that can cause fatigue, weakness, and swelling of lower extremities, as well as hair loss.
- ➤ I encourage my patients to consume enough liquids between their meals to satisfy their thirst and prevent dehydration. Six to eight 8-ounce glasses of noncaloric, decaffeinated liquids are recommended per day. But do not drink immediately before, during, or after meals. Separation of liquids and solids is recommended to maintain a feeling of fullness. If you drink while you are eating it can dissolve the food and leave you feeling empty, which can cause overeating.

I hope that you will enjoy the fabulous recipes in this unique and exciting cookbook designed especially for you. The more you use it, the closer you'll come to knowing that you cannot only eat right, but also eat well, as you strive to attain your weight loss goals.

Meredith Urban-Skuro, MS, RD, CDN received a master of science degree in clinical nutrition from New York University. She has worked with the bariatric population since 2001 and has written numerous book chapters and journal articles on nutrition and dietary guidelines for the bariatric patient. Meredith has been guest speaker at the American Society for Metabolic and Bariatric Surgery (ASMBS) and the International Federation for the Surgery of Obesity and Metabolic Disorders.

How to Use This Cookbook

At THE BOTTOM of each recipe, you'll find specific guidelines for preparation and a recommended serving size for every stage of the eating programs for gastric sleeve, gastric bypass, Lap-Band, and BPD-DS patients. We have also included preparation and serving suggestions for everyone else (referred to as "Others"—people who have not had weight-reduction surgery). These guidelines are listed under the following headings: *Gastric Sleeve and Bypass, Lap-Band, BPD-DS*, and *Others*.

In addition, you'll find a nutritional analysis breakdown below the guideline information. It includes calories, protein, fat, carbohydrates, cholesterol, fiber, and sodium. All analyses are based on an average portion size (*Others'* portions). Obviously, if you are a postsurgical patient, for the first few months you'll be eating smaller portions than the analyzed amounts, so you will be taking in even fewer calories, and less fat, carbs, cholesterol, fiber, and sodium per recipe. (*Note: We rarely add salt while we're cooking; that's why most recipes list "Salt and pepper to taste." Be aware that the salt and pepper you add will not be reflected in the nutritional analyses.*)

You have probably discussed a food program with your doctor and nutritionist. Please check with your doctor and nutritionist to make sure they agree with these guidelines. The guidelines we are using were suggested by my nutritionist. Of course, she stressed that people's tolerances vary greatly; so while we may recommend an ingredient or a recipe as being appropriate for a specific stage of your diet progression, only you will know what foods you can tolerate and when you can best tolerate them.

This book is based on my eating adventures and experiences after my Lap-Band surgery. I was very lucky and had almost no digestion problems from the get-go. In fact, I found that I had fewer problems after surgery than I had had before. But I realize that's not always the case. Some people are very sensitive to specific foods after bariatric surgery. If that's the case for you, you may want to delay trying certain recipes until later in your eating program.

For example, if you find that you are unable to comfortably digest something like beef until Week 12 or 16 but you love our recipe, which says you can eat it after Week 8, try preparing the recipe with chicken, turkey, or fish instead. You'll notice that, because many people have problems with gas or bloating from certain vegetables, maybe you'll have to wait until after Week 8 to eat recipes that include them. But, if you're like me, you can eat virtually all vegetables from the very beginning.

Don't be afraid to be flexible. Try adding new foods gradually. This book is all about making the program work for you.

Hints for Food Preparation, Cooking, and Eating

SUGGESTED KITCHEN EQUIPMENT

You will need the following:

A food processor and/or a blender

A mini-processor and/or a mini-chopper

Nonstick cookware

8 (4-ounce) ramekins

A 4-quart Dutch oven or soup pot

I also recommend these optional kitchen toys:

A Spiralizer for making zasta (zucchini pasta) among other stuff

An immersion or stick blender for pureeing soups and sauces

A microwave oven is a real convenience, as it allows you to cook in larger quantities, puree or blend, store in the refrigerator or freezer, and then reheat.

TIPS FOR COOKING

Here are some things that I have discovered through my cooking experiences that may help you:

➤ Spices, herbs, garlic, hot sauce, and mustard have almost no calories and they can make all the difference between being miserable and being satisfied. Don't be afraid to add curry powder to yogurt as a base to puree chicken. Garlic (and we use a lot of it) can liven up just about anything.

➤ When a recipe calls for artificial sweetener, do not use aspartame (Equal or NutraSweet) if you're cooking or baking—aspartame breaks down when heated. Use Splenda or Truvia. (You can use aspartame for noncooked dishes.)

➤ If we haven't specified a low-sodium product but you find one in your market, go ahead and try it. That this will bring the sodium level in the nutritional analysis down—which is ideal for just about anyone.

➤ As someone who used to cook with lots of butter and olive oil, I was amazed that switching to cooking sprays didn't really change the taste of my favorite dishes. But I did find that the flavor of the cooking sprays does often make a difference. That's why in most recipes I specify which cooking spray to use—butter-flavored, olive oil, or canola oil.

► In those rare recipes in which butter or margarine is necessary, I use a little bit of butter or light margarine. Here's a hint: even though the manufacturers of Benecol margarine and other "heart-healthy" lighter margarines (which have half the calories of butter or regular margarine) recommend that they not be used for cooking, you can use them for quick sautéing, such as making eggs.

► Most cooks have their own personal favorite ingredient. In my case, I cannot cook without some brand of concentrated chicken or beef broth (such as Bovril or Bovrite, Knorr, and Campbell's). I don't mix it with water. I add a teaspoon or two straight from the jar to recipes for maximum flavor. *Note: you can order Bovril and Bovrite at Amazon.com.*

► When a recipe calls for eggs, I generally use an egg substitute (such as Egg Beaters or Better'n Eggs). When I need whipped egg whites, I usually use egg-substitute whites (such as AllWhites). But in a few instances—for example, when I make flans or custardlike dishes—I do find that only whole large eggs or whole egg yolks will work. By the way, egg substitutes are pasteurized, so using them in uncooked recipes is not a health hazard.

► When a recipe calls for fresh lemon or lime juice, heat the fruit in the microwave on HIGH for 10 seconds. It makes it easier to juice.

► Why reinvent the wheel? Commercially prepared brands of fat-free, sugar-free ice cream, sherbet, and frozen yogurt are as good, if not better, than any that we could devise (and we tried). Of course, they taste terrific when you top them or layer them with one of our dessert sauces. But be careful: many of these diet desserts are made with sugar alcohols (sorbitol and mannitol, for example), which can cause gas, diarrhea, and bloating.

► I've found that freezing and storing excess food in ice cube trays lets me easily defrost and reheat small portions later on.

TIPS FOR EATING

► Here's a hint that's really worked for me: since you can only eat a small amount at each meal, use a salad plate instead of a dinner plate, and a salad fork and teaspoon instead of a dinner fork and soup spoon. You may also want to invest in some small dessert-size bowls, which are perfect for soups and purees.

► If you need to slow down your eating, try using chopsticks—and remember to chew each mouthful twenty-five times (Meredith made me write that).

► When eating with others who can have regular-size portions, try to pace yourself to match the other person so that you don't finish eating before he or she does.

► When pureeing your food, if you find that the puree is too dry, add a little water, milk, stock, or broth.

TIPS FOR DRINKING

➤ At my first meeting with my nutritionist, she stressed how important it was that I learn to eat without drinking any liquids immediately before, after, or during my meals. This was one of the toughest things for me to do, as I was the type of person who would tell the waiter at a restaurant to just leave the water pitcher on the table.

➤ I assumed that she stressed this "no drinking rule" because my food capacity was so diminished she did not want me to fill up on liquids. Wrong! She explained that drinking liquids with meals makes the food wash down more easily, so you may actually end up eating more than you should. Obviously, this will defeat the purpose of your surgery.

➤ But even though you can't drink liquids with meals, you do need to drink at least six to eight 8-ounce glasses of water or other noncaloric liquid each day. I keep a glass of diet iced tea or a bottle of water within grabbing distance at all times (except mealtimes, of course).

GENERAL TIPS FOR JUST GETTING ALONG

➤ Since the first few months of soft food allows you no opportunity for chewing, try chewing sugar-free gum. Before I took this advice (offered by my brother-in-law), I found myself clenching and grinding my teeth. Even if you are not a gum-chewer (and I wasn't), keep it handy and chew a piece when no one else is around. Meredith disagrees with this so I'm including her warning: *chewing gum can cause lots of gas.*

➤ Here's an interesting personal discovery I made that may help you, too: Meredith had warned me that after surgery I might have problems with constipation. She suggested that I take a daily fiber supplement, such as Citrucel or Benefiber, and I found that sometimes it worked and sometimes it didn't. Then I had an idea: instead of fiber (after all, I was getting plenty of fiber from fruits and vegetables), what if I took one 400 IU softgel of vitamin E every day? I don't know if it was the vitamin E itself or the tiny amount of soybean oil it was suspended in that was the magic ingredient—but it worked!

Stocking Your Pantry and Refrigerator

IF YOU'RE LIKE me, you get really annoyed when you want to make a certain recipe, only to find that you're missing one ingredient. That's why I thought it would be really handy to provide you with a pantry list of the basic essentials, plus some of the specialty ingredients that we used to create these recipes.

I found that having a variety of flavors to choose from made it easier to stick to my eating program even after the restriction period was over. To achieve that in everyday cooking, you need to stock your pantry and refrigerator with spices, herbs, and condiments. Here are my suggestions:

PANTRY

Anchovy paste: We don't use this ingredient that often, but when a recipe calls for it, nothing else will really do. *Note: this is very high in sodium.*

Artificial sweetener: Don't cook with aspartame (Equal or NutraSweet) because it breaks down under high temperatures. It is perfectly fine for adding to hot beverages, sprinkling on fruit, or mixing into noncooked recipes. For cooking, Splenda or Truvia works better. Sweet'N Low also makes a very good brown-sugar artificial sweetener.

Asian sauces and oils: At one time many of these sauces were considered exotic, but now just about every supermarket stocks them. They are highly distinctive in flavor, each adding an individual kick to the recipes in which they appear:

Asian chili paste with garlic
green curry sauce
light soy sauce

red chili paste
red curry sauce
sesame oil

Broth : Fat-free, low-sodium canned chicken, beef, and vegetable broth are absolute necessities for this cookbook. They provide both flavor and moisture without adding unnecessary fat or salt. But stock has twice the calories that broth does, so I use broth, then add a teaspoon of concentrated broth, if necessary.

Capers: Capers have a bright, almost metallic taste that really perks up simple dishes. They are bottled in brine, so you may want to rinse them off to reduce the sodium.

Clam juice or broth: A perfect low-fat liquid base for seafood soups and sauces. There are a number of good bottled brands, such as Doxee or Look's Atlantic Brand.

Cocoa powder, unsweetened: The key ingredient in low-fat hot cocoa, chocolate sauces, and desserts.

Concentrated broth: This is perfect for adding more beef or chicken flavor to sauces, soups, or stews. It's also more convenient than opening a whole can of broth for a recipe that only requires a couple of spoonfuls. Bovril, Bovrite, Knorr, and College Inn make very good concentrated broth in both chicken and beef flavors. You can order Chicken Bovril and Beef Bovrite at online retailers, such as Amazon.com. *Note: Concentrated broth is high in sodium, but some stores carry reduced-sodium alternatives.*

Cooking spray: There are a lot of different brands available and I've found that most of them offer an easy, fat-free way to fry or sauté foods without adding oil. I always keep three flavors on hand—butter, canola oil, and olive oil.

Dried mushrooms: If you want to add a really intense mushroom flavor to soups or stews, throw in some of these just as they are. For quicker-cooking dishes, I soak them in boiling water, then strain the water and use both the softened mushrooms and the liquid. You can find plain white dried mushrooms, as well as more exciting ones, such as dried shiitakes, dried morels, dried chanterelles, and dried mixed exotic mushrooms in most supermarkets.

Dried spices and herbs: Keeping a variety of these dried and/or ground flavorings on hand is a must for the recipes in this cookbook. You probably already have a lot of them, so it just means a bit of filling in.

allspice	cream of tartar	onion flakes
basil	cumin	minced onion
cardamom	curry powder	oregano
cayenne pepper	dill	paprika (sweet and hot)
celery flakes	fennel seeds	parsley
celery salt	garam masala	red pepper flakes
celery seed	garlic powder	saffron threads
chili powder	ginger	steak rub seasoning
cinnamon	lemon-pepper	tarragon
cloves (whole and ground)	mint	thyme
coriander	nutmeg	turmeric

Evaporated skim or fat-free milk: This is a wonderful ingredient when you want a soup or a sauce to be slightly richer or thicker, but don't want to add carbs or calories. It reduces down very nicely and caramelizes beautifully.

Flavor extracts: These are lots fun to experiment with, and they don't add any extra calories. We found a number of sites on the web that offer an incredible variety—for example, www.Penzeys.com and www.spicebarn.com. Of course, you'll want vanilla, but we also suggest coconut and almond.

Garlic: To me, you can never have too much garlic—but don't worry, I did use restraint when I developed these recipes. I always keep a bunch of fresh heads of garlic around, and when I need some, I smack a few garlic cloves with the flat of a knife, then peel and chop them. If you prefer to use a garlic press or mince them in a mini-chopper, feel free. (*Here's Michele's hint: to take the garlic smell off your fingers, hold the blade of a metal knife in your fingers—both hands—and run it under cold water. It's magic!*) Garlic powder, dried or fresh minced garlic, or dried roasted garlic are all available at most supermarkets.

Horseradish: Talk about pungent! This is one of the best perker-uppers we know. It goes especially well with creamy sauces. I use prepared, bottled white horseradish and drain it well before adding it to recipes.

Juices: While fresh citrus juices are preferable, sometimes you just don't have fresh fruit in the house or you don't want to cut up a whole lemon or lime just to squeeze out a spoonful. I always keep bottles of orange, lemon, and lime juices as well as small cans of tomato juice in my pantry.

Mayonnaise: Nothing takes the place of mayo in sauces and cold salads. That's why it's great that all of the manufacturers now offer light and fat-free versions. We tried a lot of different ones and do prefer the light (25 calories per tablespoon) over the fat-free (10 calories per tablespoon)—it's a matter of taste.

Mustard: While this condiment is quite pungent straight from the jar, it mellows out deliciously during the cooking process. We use both Dijon and whole-grain mustard in our recipes.

Roasted red peppers: Sure, you can char and peel fresh peppers, but why bother? Many traditional Spanish-accented recipes call for bottled roasted red peppers.

Sauces: There are a number of condiment sauces that can really liven up a recipe. I always keep some brand of hot sauce as well as Worcestershire sauce and chili sauce on hand.

Shallots: Fresh shallots are probably the subtlest member of the onion family. I always keep a bag of them in stock. Shallots are so convenient to use—I admit, sometimes when a recipe calls for a small amount of onion, instead of peeling a whole big onion, I use a couple of shallot cloves instead.

Soy nuts: After you're through the soft-food stage and you want a bit of crunch, try toasted soy nuts. I grind them in my mini-processor and use them as a crunchy topping, or use them instead of breadcrumbs with egg substitute to make a low-carb coating for fish, pork, or chicken. They are very high in protein. You can find them in some supermarkets and all health food shops.

Tomatoes, canned: Although some recipes call for fresh tomatoes, in many cases we've stipulated using different types of canned tomatoes. Here are some suggestions:

crushed tomatoes with juice, 28-ounce can

diced tomatoes, 14.5-ounce can

Italian-style plum tomatoes, 28-ounce can

stewed tomatoes, 14.5-ounce can

sun-dried tomato paste in a tube

tomato paste in a tube

tomato paste, 6-ounce can

tomato sauce, 8- or 14.5-ounce can

tomato puree, 14.5- or 28-ounce can

whole peeled tomatoes, 28-ounce can

Unsweetened low-fat or light coconut milk: This is another one of those surprising ingredients that we found when we were looking for something that would add thickness and richness to a dish without adding a lot of fat or calories. Don't worry if you're not a big fan of coconut; the flavor is very subtle.

Wasabi: Although once referred to as Japanese mustard, wasabi is really a type of ground horseradish. You can buy it in powder form and mix it with water, but I buy it as a paste in a handy tube.

Wines: I know that most food experts say that you shouldn't cook with any wine you wouldn't drink. Well, call me a philistine, but if I don't have an opened bottle of wine around, I use commercial brands of cooking wine. You'll need dry white wine, dry red wine, dry sherry, and dry vermouth.

Vinegars: I love having a variety of vinegars to play with. Our recipes call for balsamic, cider, and red wine vinegars, as well as Asian rice vinegar. But why stop there? Try raspberry vinegar or sherry pepper vinegar, too.

REFRIGERATOR

Artificial butter spray: I always keep a bottle of I Can't Believe It's Not Butter spray in my fridge for spritzing on steamed vegetables or mixing into mashed cauliflower.

Cheddar cheese, low-fat: This is just fine for cooking purposes, and some is even okay for eating plain. Cabot makes a 50 percent low-fat Cheddar that is fine for cooking or eating, but I will use their 75 percent low-fat Cheddar only for cooking.

Cream cheese, fat-free: Although you probably wouldn't want to eat this plain, as a cooking ingredient it adds a luscious, creamy richness to a number of our recipes.

Egg substitute: When a recipe calls for eggs, I generally use egg substitute (such as Egg Beaters or Better'n Eggs). When I need whipped egg whites, I usually use egg substitute whites (such as AllWhites or other brands).

Fresh herbs: I love using fresh herbs, especially in quick-cooking recipes. Since most recipes just call for small amounts, I freeze my fresh herbs in resealable plastic bags (with all the air pushed out), and I just use them as needed. *Don't defrost frozen herbs before using—they turn black and slimy.* Here are the ones I like to have on hand:

basil	rosemary
chive	sage
cilantro	tarragon
mint	thyme
parsley	

Fresh mushrooms: My mother once told me that I buy mushrooms the way other people by bread and milk. I absolutely love them. Fresh, firm white or cremini mushrooms have always been a staple in my house. Meredith did ask me to warn you that some people have gas problems with mushrooms.

Hot peppers: Michele introduced me to cooking with hot peppers, but I admit: I'm still a little timid. So, if you're like me, since most of the heat is in the seeds, make sure that you scrape off all the seeds. (You may also want to wear kitchen gloves while handling hot peppers, as the hot pepper oil can stick to your skin and won't wash off easily.) Look for small, firm jalapeño or serrano peppers.

Mozzarella, part skim: This is great for cooking Italian-style dishes when you want that melted, stretchy cheese experience. I even use it in omelets.

Parmesan: As far as we can tell, there is no hard grating cheese that is available in a low-fat version. Oh well. We justify including this tasty grated cheese by not using too much in any recipe.

Ricotta, fat-free: I don't particularly like this for eating plain, but it works very well as an ingredient in our recipes. It's soft, creamy, and blends deliciously with herbs.

Sour cream, fat-free: This is a perfect substitute for full-fat sour cream when it's used as we do, as an ingredient in recipes. It adds a very creamy, rich taste and texture without adding fat.

Swiss-type cheese, low-fat: There are a number of nutty-tasting cheeses with holes that we generically refer to as Swiss. If you have a good cheese store or a well-stocked supermarket, you can usually find low-fat or Lite Dammer, Gruyère, or domestic Swiss.

Yogurt, plain, fat-free: An absolute essential in making these recipes. And for eating by itself, I actually prefer it to the whole-fat or flavored yogurts—I mix a couple of spoonfuls of one of our fruit sauces into it and it tastes incredible.

Breakfast and Brunch

Breakfast and brunch dishes to wake your taste buds

EVEN THOUGH YOU are eating less, it is still important to eat breakfast. In the first weeks after surgery, when you are on a soft diet, remember that protein should be a key component of your meal. That's why we've included recipes for savory scrambled eggs and omelets that taste just as delicious pureed (if necessary) as they do whole.

Virtually all of these dishes use egg substitute to reduce your calorie intake. If you're careful not to overcook them, I think you can barely tell the difference between these scrambled eggs or omelets and ones made with whole eggs.

All of these recipes already call for truly delectable combinations of ingredients, but we encourage you to go ahead and experiment. Instead of broccoli, use asparagus or spinach. Play with different spices and herbs. And if you don't feel ready for the firmer texture of an omelet or simply prefer scrambled eggs to omelets, go ahead and scramble all the ingredients together. If you're cooking for just one, eggs and omelets are some of the easiest and most satisfying foods to make in an individual portion—simply use one quarter of each of the ingredients.

Best of all, there's no need to wait for breakfast to enjoy these tasty meals. I make many of these dishes for lunch and even for light dinners on a regular basis. You'll also find a number of other dishes in other sections of this cookbook that work well for breakfast or brunch. Try the Zucchini Flan with Quick Tomato Sauce (page 53), the Crustless Spinach and Cheese Quiche (page 47), or any of the incredibly luscious fruit smoothies in the Sweet Indulgences section (pages 179–181).

You'll find that breakfast and brunch can be just as interesting and satisfying as every other meal—so enjoy.

Note: The nutritional analyses are based on average portion size (*Others'* portions).

Broccoli and Cheese Omelet

This is a delicious twist on the basic cheese omelet. The broccoli and shallots add a subtle sweetness to the nutty taste of Swiss.

1 cup chopped broccoli florets
¼ cup minced shallots
1 tablespoon water
Butter-flavored cooking spray
1 cup egg substitute
4 ounces low-fat Swiss, diced
Salt and pepper to taste

1. Mix broccoli, shallots, and water in a small microwaveable bowl. Cover with plastic wrap and microwave on HIGH for 3½ minutes, or until broccoli is soft.
2. *To make each omelet:* In a medium lidded skillet, heat cooking spray over medium heat until hot but not smoking. Pour in ¼ cup egg substitute and swirl to coat bottom of pan.
3. Place 1 ounce diced cheese on one half of omelet and cover cheese with 2 tablespoons of broccoli mixture. Fold unfilled half of omelet over filling, lower heat, cover pan, and cook for 1 to 2 minutes, or until cheese melts.
4. Slide omelet onto plate and keep warm. Re-spray skillet and repeat for all remaining omelets. Add salt and pepper to taste.

Makes 4 omelets

► **Cooking Tip:** For individual omelets, beat ¼ cup egg substitute with 1 teaspoon water until frothy.

SERVING GUIDELINES

► **FOR GASTRIC SLEEVE AND BYPASS:**
Week 1: Liquid diet.
Weeks 2–4: Puree ½–1 omelet until smooth.
Weeks 5–7: Chop ½–1 omelet.
Weeks 8+: Serve ½–1 omelet as is.

► **FOR BPD-DS:**
Week 1: Liquid diet.
Weeks 2–3: Puree ½–1 omelet until smooth.
Weeks 4+: Serve 1 omelet as is.

► **FOR LAP-BAND:**
Week 1: Liquid diet.
Weeks 2–4: Puree ½–1 omelet until smooth.
Weeks 5–7: Chop ½–1 omelet.
Weeks 8+: Serve ½ omelet as is.

► **FOR OTHERS:**
Serve 1 omelet as is.

Calories: 122, **Protein:** 15 g, **Fat:** 4 g, **Carbohydrates:** 5 g, **Cholesterol:** 15 mg, **Fiber:** 0 g, **Sodium:** 169 mg

Omelet Italiano

I like to describe this omelet as a brunch pizza without the crust. And, just as with pizza, you can experiment and change the fillings: try bell peppers instead of mushrooms or Canadian bacon instead of sausage. But remember, that will change the nutritional numbers, too.

Butter-flavored cooking spray
2 low-fat turkey sausages
 (sweet Italian-style)
8 to 10 fresh mushrooms, thinly sliced
½ cup chopped onion
1 cup chopped ripe plum tomatoes
2 teaspoons dried basil
1 cup egg substitute
4 teaspoons water
4 ounces grated part-skim
 mozzarella cheese
Salt and pepper to taste

1. In a large nonstick lidded skillet, heat cooking spray over medium heat until hot but not smoking. While skillet is heating, remove sausage meat from casings; then brown it, breaking up lumps, for 2 minutes.
2. Add mushrooms and onion and brown them, stirring, for 2 minutes.
3. Stir in tomatoes and basil, lower heat, and cook, covered, for 3 minutes, or until tomatoes are softened.
4. Remove sausage-tomato mixture from skillet and keep warm.
5. *To make each omelet:* In a small bowl, combine ¼ cup egg substitute with 1 teaspoon water and beat well.
6. Heat medium lidded skillet over medium heat until hot but not smoking. Pour in egg substitute and swirl pan until entire bottom is covered. Place 1 ounce cheese on one half of egg and top with 3 tablespoons of sausage mixture.
7. Fold other side of omelet over filling, lower heat, and cook, covered, for 2 minutes, or until cheese melts.
8. Slide omelet onto plate and keep warm. Re-spray pan and repeat for all remaining omelets. Add salt and pepper to taste.

Makes 4 servings

SERVING GUIDELINES

► **FOR GASTRIC SLEEVE AND BYPASS:**
 Week 1: Liquid diet.
 Weeks 2–4: Puree ½–1 omelet until smooth.
 Weeks 5–7: Chop ½–1 omelet.
 Weeks 8+: Serve ½–1 omelet as is.

► **FOR BPD-DS:**
 Week 1: Liquid diet.
 Weeks 2–3: Puree ½–1 omelet until smooth.
 Weeks 4+: Serve 1 omelet as is.

► **FOR LAP-BAND:**
 Week 1: Liquid diet.
 Weeks 2–4: Puree ½–1 omelet until smooth.
 Weeks 5–7: Chop ½–1 omelet.
 Weeks 8+: Serve ½ omelet as is.

► **FOR OTHERS:**
 Serve 1 omelet as is.

Calories: 193, **Protein:** 19 g, **Fat:** 9 g, **Carbohydrates:** 7 g, **Cholesterol:** 43 mg, **Fiber:** 1 g, **Sodium:** 707 mg

Omelet à la Quebec

I first tasted this delicious turkey and mushroom omelet on a trip to Canada and made it part of my cooking repertoire as soon as we returned. Of course, Michele and I adapted it for this book, but it tastes just as good.

8 ounces fresh mushrooms, thinly sliced
5 teaspoons water
4 ounces (4 thin slices) cooked turkey breast, torn into small pieces
1 cup egg substitute
Butter-flavored cooking spray
4 ounces low-fat Cheddar cheese, diced
Salt and pepper to taste

1. Place mushrooms and 1 tablespoon water in a small microwaveable bowl, cover with plastic wrap, and microwave on HIGH for 3 minutes. Mix turkey pieces into cooked mushrooms.
2. *To make each omelet:* In a separate bowl, beat ¼ cup egg substitute with 1 teaspoon water.
3. In a medium nonstick lidded skillet, heat cooking spray over medium heat until hot but not smoking. Pour in ¼ cup egg substitute–water mixture, swirling pan until entire bottom is covered.
4. Scatter 1 ounce cheese on one half of omelet and cover cheese with 2 tablespoons of mushroom-turkey mixture.
5. Fold unfilled half of omelet over filling; lower heat, cover, and cook for 1 to 2 minutes, or until cheese melts.
6. Slide omelet out of pan and keep warm. Add salt and pepper to taste. Re-spray skillet and repeat for all remaining omelets.

Makes 4 servings

SERVING GUIDELINES

▶ **FOR GASTRIC SLEEVE AND BYPASS:**
   Week 1: Liquid diet.
   Weeks 2–4: Puree ½–1 omelet until smooth.
   Weeks 5–7: Chop ½–1 omelet.
   Weeks 8+: Serve ½–1 omelet as is.

▶ **FOR BPD-DS:**
   Week 1: Liquid diet.
   Weeks 2–3: Puree ½–1 omelet until smooth.
   Weeks 4+: Serve 1 omelet as is.

▶ **FOR LAP-BAND:**
   Week 1: Liquid diet.
   Weeks 2–4: Puree ½–1 omelet until smooth.
   Weeks 5–7: Chop ½–1 omelet.
   Weeks 8+: Serve ½ omelet as is.

▶ **FOR OTHERS:**
   Serve 1 omelet as is.

Calories: 126, **Protein:** 23 g, **Fat:** 2 g, **Carbohydrates:** 3 g, **Cholesterol:** 20 mg, **Fiber:** 2 g, **Sodium:** 348 mg

Scrambled Eggs with Ham and Cheese

Yes, there is a way to eat the all-American favorite breakfast combination and still eat the way you should. Here it is.

1 cup egg substitute
1 tablespoon water
4 ounces low-fat Cheddar cheese, diced
4 ounces low-fat sliced ham,
    finely minced
Butter-flavored cooking spray
Salt and pepper to taste

1. In a small bowl, beat egg substitute with water until frothy. Stir in cheese and ham.
2. In a medium nonstick skillet, heat cooking spray over medium heat until hot but not smoking. Pour in egg mixture, stirring constantly for 1 to 2 minutes, or until eggs form small curds that are soft but not runny and cheese melts. Add salt and pepper to taste.

Makes 4 servings

SERVING GUIDELINES

▶ **FOR GASTRIC SLEEVE AND BYPASS:**
    Week 1: Liquid diet.
    Weeks 2+: Serve ¼–½ cup scrambled eggs as is.

▶ **FOR BPD-DS:**
    Week 1: Liquid diet.
    Weeks 2+: Serve ½ cup scrambled eggs as is.

▶ **FOR LAP-BAND:**
    Week 1: Liquid diet.
    Weeks 2+: Serve ¼–½ cup scrambled eggs as is.

▶ **FOR OTHERS:**
    Serve ½ cup scrambled eggs as is.

Calories: 108, **Protein:** 18 g, **Fat:** 3 g, **Carbohydrates:** 2 g, **Cholesterol:** 20 mg, **Fiber:** 0 g, **Sodium:** 618 mg

Chicken Livers and Scrambled Eggs

This is my ultimate comfort food, a seemingly indulgent but healthy dish—and it's perfect for anyone who's cutting back on carbs. It's great for breakfast, brunch, or even a light supper.

Butter-flavored cooking spray
1 large sweet onion, quartered and sliced
8 ounces fresh mushrooms, sliced
1 pound chicken livers, rinsed
4 large eggs, or 1 cup egg substitute
  lightly beaten with 1 teaspoon water
¼ teaspoon curry powder
Salt and pepper to taste

1. Spray a large skillet with cooking spray and heat over medium heat until it shimmers.
2. Add onion and mushrooms, cooking until onion softens and mushrooms give up their liquid, 4 to 6 minutes.
3. While onions and mushrooms are cooking, trim connective tissue and roughly chop chicken livers.
4. Stir chicken livers into skillet and cook until they just start to brown, 5 to 7 minutes.
5. Mix eggs with curry powder and pour into skillet, stirring to coat livers, onion, and mushrooms. Cook, stirring constantly, for 1 to 2 minutes, or until eggs form small curds that are soft but not runny.

Makes 4 servings

SERVING GUIDELINES

- **FOR GASTRIC SLEEVE AND BYPASS:**
  Week 1: Liquid diet.
  Weeks 2–3: Puree 2 ounces cooked chicken livers and eggs.
  Weeks 4+: Serve 2 ounces cooked chicken livers and eggs as is.

- **FOR BPD-DS:**
  Week 1: Liquid diet.
  Weeks 2–3: Puree 2 ounces cooked chicken livers and eggs.
  Weeks 4+: Serve 2–4 ounces cooked chicken livers and eggs as is.

- **FOR LAP-BAND:**
  Week 1: Liquid diet.
  Weeks 2–3: Puree 2 ounces cooked chicken livers and eggs.
  Weeks 4+: Serve 2 ounces cooked chicken livers and eggs as is.

- **FOR OTHERS:**
  Serve 4 ounces cooked chicken livers and eggs as is.

Calories: 251, **Protein:** 29 g, **Fat:** 9 g, **Carbohydrates:** 11 g, **Cholesterol:** 186 mg, **Fiber:** 1 g, **Sodium:** 81 mg

Vegetable Frittata

Whenever I'm having company for brunch, I make this dish. It's a real crowd-pleaser and much easier than serving omelets for a group.

1 cup egg substitute
2 tablespoons water
Butter-flavored cooking spray
1 medium zucchini, cut into ½-inch cubes (about 1 cup)
1 cup diced fresh mushrooms
½ cup thinly sliced onion
1 small bell pepper, seeded and cut into ½-inch cubes (about ½ cup)
½ cup grated Parmesan cheese
Salt and pepper to taste

1. In medium bowl, beat egg substitute with water until well mixed.
2. In large nonstick lidded skillet, heat cooking spray over medium heat until hot but not smoking. Sauté zucchini, mushrooms, onion, and bell pepper for 3 to 5 minutes, or until lightly browned and softened.
3. Pour egg substitute over vegetable mixture. Lower heat, cover skillet, and cook for 1 to 2 minutes, or until set.
4. Sprinkle cheese on top of frittata and place under preheated broiler for 1 to 2 minutes, or until cheese browns. Add salt and pepper to taste.

Makes 4 servings

SERVING GUIDELINES

► **FOR GASTRIC SLEEVE AND BYPASS:**
Week 1: Liquid diet.
Weeks 2–3: Puree ¼–½ cup frittata until smooth.
Weeks 4–7: Chop ¼–½ cup frittata.
Weeks 8+: Serve ¼–½ cup frittata as is.

► **FOR BPD-DS:**
Week 1: Liquid diet.
Weeks 2–3: Puree ½ cup frittata until smooth.
Weeks 4+: Serve ¼–½ cup frittata as is.

► **FOR LAP-BAND:**
Week 1: Liquid diet.
Weeks 2–4: Puree ¼–½ cup frittata until smooth.
Weeks 4–7: Chop ¼–½ cup frittata.
Weeks 8+: Serve ¼–½ cup frittata as is.

► **FOR OTHERS:**
Serve ¼ frittata as is.

Calories: 108, **Protein:** 13 g, **Fat:** 4 g, **Carbohydrates:** 6 g, **Cholesterol:** 10 mg, **Fiber:** 1 g, **Sodium:** 335 mg

Deviled Egg Salad

Tangy and slightly spicy, this is a nice change for breakfast or lunch. You could even pack it for lunch or a snack at work.

4 medium eggs
2 tablespoons low-fat mayonnaise
1 teaspoon dried minced onion
2 teaspoons Dijon mustard
2 teaspoons sweet or hot paprika
Salt and pepper to taste
Hot sauce to taste (optional)

1. Place eggs in a small pot, add water to cover, and bring to a boil over high heat. Cook for 18 minutes.
2. Run cold water over eggs for 1 to 2 minutes, or until eggs are cool enough to handle.
3. Peel eggs and cut into quarters.
4. Place eggs, mayonnaise, dried onion, mustard, and paprika in a food processor or mini-chopper and pulse for 15 seconds, or until almost smooth. Add salt, pepper, and hot sauce (if using) to taste.

Makes 4 servings

SERVING GUIDELINES

► **FOR GASTRIC SLEEVE AND BYPASS:**
Week 1: Liquid diet.
Weeks 2+: Serve ¼ cup egg salad as is.

► **FOR BPD-DS:**
Week 1: Liquid diet.
Weeks 2+: Serve ¼ cup egg salad as is.

► **FOR LAP-BAND:**
Week 1: Liquid diet.
Weeks 2+: Serve ¼ cup egg salad as is.

► **FOR OTHERS:**
Serve ¼ egg salad as is.

Calories: 95, **Protein:** 7 g, **Fat:** 6 g, **Carbohydrates:** 4 g, **Cholesterol:** 213 mg, **Fiber:** 0 g, **Sodium:** 148 mg

Soup It Up

Everlovin' spoonfuls for every season

WHEN MEREDITH FIRST showed me the guideline menus suggested for the first weeks after surgery, I was pleased to see that they included soup. I love soup. But not the kind that comes in cans. I love homemade soups, and I bet you will, too.

Some of our soup recipes are designed to be eaten as purees; all others taste great pureed but are equally good when you serve them just the way you cook them—thick with the textures of different chopped ingredients.

In this section, we offer you a fantastic selection of soups—smooth, cold summer soups; satisfying meal-in-a-bowl soups; even rich chowders and creamed soups. There are vegetable-based soups, chicken- and turkey-based soups, plus a lot of wonderful seafood soups. And they are all high in protein, low in calories, and low in carbohydrates.

It took a lot of testing and ingenuity, but we came up with a variety of ways to add creaminess or richness to many of our soup recipes. Using unsweetened light coconut milk or evaporated skim milk, we added thickness without adding distinctive flavor. Plain, fat-free yogurt or sour cream allowed us to add tangy creaminess to other recipes. And how did we make a full-bodied chowder without potatoes? We discovered that if we cook cauliflower very soft, cube some of it and mash some more, then add it, we got just the result we were looking for.

So, why relegate soup to just the beginning of a meal? Some of our soups are meals in themselves— they make great light dinners. Or, if you have access to a microwave at work, why not make your favorite recipe ahead of time and brown-bag some homemade soup for lunch? Even if you don't have a microwave, bring in one of our cold soups. Soups also make terrifically satisfying snacks—you know, those healthy snacks that we're allowed to have once or twice a day.

And, yes, we even offer a version of Mom's chicken soup—it's called Mother-in-Law Soup—I guess 'cause she uses a lot of garlic to keep her precious son from wanting to get too amorous.

Note: The nutritional analyses are based on an average portion size (*Others'* portions).

Bengali Chicken and Vegetable Soup

Chicken soup with an exotic accent: thickened with vegetables, enriched with coconut milk, and sparked with cinnamon, ginger, and jalapeño.

1 (14-ounce) can unsweetened light coconut milk
1 medium onion, chopped
1 garlic clove, minced
¼ teaspoon dried thyme
¼ cup fresh parsley
2 whole cloves
½ teaspoon ground cinnamon
1 tablespoon finely minced fresh ginger
1 small fresh jalapeño pepper, seeded and finely chopped
1 (14.5-ounce) can fat-free, low-sodium chicken broth
½ pound skinless chicken breast, diced
½ pound cauliflower florets
½ pound broccoli florets
1 large carrot, sliced
Salt and pepper to taste

1. In a large soup pot, combine coconut milk, onion, garlic, thyme, parsley, cloves, cinnamon, ginger, and jalapeño. Bring to a simmer over medium heat and let cook, uncovered, stirring occasionally, for 15 to 20 minutes, or until thickened. Remove whole cloves.
2. Stir in chicken broth, chicken, cauliflower, broccoli, and carrot. Cover pot and simmer over low heat for 1 hour. Add salt and pepper to taste.

Makes 4 servings

SERVING GUIDELINES

▶ **FOR GASTRIC SLEEVE AND BYPASS:**
Week 1: Liquid diet.
Weeks 2–4: Puree ½ cup soup.
Weeks 5+: Serve ½–1 cup soup as is.

▶ **FOR BPD-DS:**
Weeks 1: Liquid diet.
Weeks 2+: Serve ½–1 cup soup as is.

▶ **FOR LAP-BAND:**
Week 1: Liquid diet.
Weeks 2–4: Puree ½ cup soup.
Weeks 5+: Serve ½–1 cup soup as is.

▶ **FOR OTHERS:**
Serve 1 cup soup as is.

Calories: 219, **Protein:** 17 g, **Fat:** 8 g, **Carbohydrates:** 15 g, **Cholesterol:** 33 mg, **Fiber:** 4 g, **Sodium:** 521 mg

Chicken and Mushroom Soup

This soup is like the ultimate warm hug in food form. Rich and creamy with the earthy, autumn taste of fresh and dried mushrooms, this is pure comfort in a bowl.

Butter-flavored cooking spray
1½ cups chopped onion
3 garlic cloves, minced
1 pound fresh white mushrooms,
  chopped
½ teaspoon dried tarragon
1 bay leaf
¼ teaspoon dried thyme
½ cup white wine
½ pound boneless, skinless chicken
  breast, quartered
2 (14.5-ounce) cans fat-free, low-sodium
  chicken broth
⅓ cup dried shiitake mushrooms
  (about ½ ounce)
¼ cup fat-free sour cream
Salt and pepper to taste
2 tablespoons chopped fresh chives, or
  1 tablespoon dried

1. Coat bottom of a large soup pot with cooking spray and sauté onion, garlic, and fresh mushrooms over medium heat. Cover and cook for 10 minutes, stirring occasionally.
2. Add tarragon, bay leaf, thyme, and wine, stirring and scraping bottom of pot to loosen browned bits.
3. Lower heat and add chicken, chicken broth, and dried mushrooms. Cover and simmer for 30 minutes.
4. Discard bay leaf and stir in sour cream.
5. Puree soup in batches in a food processor until smooth. Add salt and pepper to taste, and top with chives.

Makes 4 servings

SERVING GUIDELINES

➤ **FOR GASTRIC SLEEVE AND BYPASS:**
  Week 1: Liquid diet.
  Weeks 2–4: Serve ½ cup soup as is.
  Weeks 5+: Serve ½–1 cup soup.

➤ **FOR BPD-DS:**
  Weeks 1: Liquid diet.
  Weeks 2+: Serve ½–1 cup soup as is.

➤ **FOR LAP-BAND:**
  Week 1: Liquid diet.
  Weeks 2–4: Serve ½ cup soup.
  Weeks 5+: Serve ½–1 cup soup as is.

➤ **FOR OTHERS:**
  Serve 1 cup as is.

Calories: 239, **Protein:** 22 g, **Fat:** 2 g, **Carbohydrates:** 33 g, **Cholesterol:** 35 mg, **Fiber:** 6 g, **Sodium:** 683 mg

Chicken Artichoke Soup

This recipe is a great way to use up your leftover chicken. It's incredibly easy to make but tastes like fine French cooking—smooth, rich, and sophisticated. Serve it hot or cold.

1 (14-ounce) can artichoke hearts in brine, drained well

2 ounces soft or silken tofu

3 tablespoons grated Parmesan cheese

1½ tablespoons fresh lemon juice

¾ teaspoon dried tarragon

2 teaspoons grated lemon zest

2 garlic cloves, minced

¼ teaspoon ground nutmeg

¼ teaspoon chili powder

2 cups fat-free, low-sodium chicken broth

½ pound cooked skinless, boneless chicken breast, cubed

1. Puree artichoke hearts in food processor until chunky.
2. Add all remaining ingredients and puree until smooth.
3. Pour into large pot, cover, and simmer over low heat for 10 minutes.

Makes 4 servings

SERVING GUIDELINES

► **FOR GASTRIC SLEEVE AND BYPASS:**
Week 1: Liquid diet.
Weeks 2–4: Puree ½ cup soup.
Weeks 5+: Serve ½–1 cup soup as is.

► **FOR BPD-DS:**
Weeks 1: Liquid diet.
Weeks 2+: Serve ½–1 cup soup as is.

► **FOR LAP-BAND:**
Week 1: Liquid diet.
Weeks 2–4: Puree ½ cup soup.
Weeks 5+: Serve ½–1 cup soup as is.

► **FOR OTHERS:**
Serve 1 cup soup as is.

Calories: 162, **Protein:** 22 g, **Fat:** 3 g, **Carbohydrates:** 12 g, **Cholesterol:** 47 mg, **Fiber:** 2 g, **Sodium:** 741 mg

Black Bean and Sausage Soup

Here's a hearty main dish soup that's perfect for a cold night with the family or served in mugs for a tailgating picnic.

2 (15-ounce) cans low-sodium black beans, drained and rinsed

2½ cups low-sodium chicken, beef, or turkey broth

Olive oil cooking spray

2 cups diced onion

2 garlic cloves, minced

1 teaspoon chili powder

½ teaspoon ground cumin

¼ teaspoon freshly ground black pepper

¼–½ teaspoon hot sauce

1 (16-ounce) package frozen chopped spinach or kale, thawed

8 ounces turkey kielbasa, diced

½ cup reduced-fat sour cream (optional)

1. Pour 1 cup black beans and ½ cup broth into blender. Blend until smooth.
2. Spray a large pot or Dutch oven with cooking spray and heat over medium-high heat until shimmering.
3. Sauté onion and garlic until soft but not browned, about 5 minutes.
4. Add bean puree, whole beans, remaining broth, seasonings, hot sauce, and spinach and bring to a boil. Lower heat, cover, and simmer for 15 minutes, stirring occasionally.
5. Stir in kielbasa and cook, stirring, for 5 minutes.
6. Ladle into bowls or mugs and top with sour cream, if desired.

Makes 4–8 servings

SERVING GUIDELINES

► **FOR GASTRIC SLEEVE AND BYPASS:**
Week 1: Liquid diet.
Weeks 2–3: Puree 2 ounces soup.
Weeks 4–7: Chop 2 ounces soup.
Weeks 8+: Serve 2–4 ounces soup.

► **FOR BPD-DS:**
Week 1: Liquid diet.
Weeks 2–3: Puree 2 ounces soup.
Weeks 4+: Serve 2–4 ounces soup.

► **FOR LAP-BAND:**
Week 1: Liquid diet.
Weeks 2–7: Puree 2 ounces soup.
Weeks 4–7: Chop 2 ounces soup.
Weeks 8+: Serve 2–4 ounces soup.

► **FOR OTHERS:**
Serve 1 cup soup.

Calories: 326, **Protein:** 27 g, **Fat:** 4 g, **Carbohydrates:** 44 g, **Cholesterol:** 35 mg, **Fiber:** 17 g, **Sodium:** 785 mg

Mother-in-Law Soup

You've heard of Mama's chicken soup? Well, this is the Spanish mother-in-law's version, golden with saffron and gutsy with garlic. I substituted prosciutto for the traditional Serrano ham because it's easier to find in the market.

Olive oil cooking spray
4 large garlic cloves, minced
1 ounce prosciutto, diced
1 teaspoon sweet paprika
¼ teaspoon ground cumin
¼ teaspoon freshly ground black pepper
⅛ teaspoon saffron threads
2 (14.5-ounce) cans fat-free, low-sodium chicken broth
4 large eggs
Salt to taste

1. In a large nonstick saucepan, heat cooking spray over medium-high heat until hot but not smoking. Sauté garlic for 1 minute. Add prosciutto and paprika, and sauté for 30 more seconds.
2. Stir in cumin, pepper, and saffron, add broth, and bring to a boil.
3. Cover pan, lower heat, and simmer for 20 minutes.
4. One at a time, carefully break eggs into soup and simmer for 3 minutes until whites are set. Add salt to taste. Serve soup with one poached egg per serving.

Makes 4 servings

SERVING GUIDELINES

► **FOR GASTRIC SLEEVE AND BYPASS:**
Week 1: Liquid diet.
Weeks 2–4: Puree ½ cup soup with 1 poached egg.
Weeks 5+: Serve ½–1 cup soup with 1 poached egg.

► **FOR BPD-DS:**
Weeks 1: Liquid diet.
Weeks 2+: Serve ½–1 cup soup with 1 poached egg.

► **FOR LAP-BAND:**
Week 1: Liquid diet.
Weeks 2–4: Puree ½ cup soup with 1 poached egg.
Weeks 5+: Serve ½–1 cup with 1 poached egg.

► **FOR OTHERS:**
Serve 1 cup soup with 1 poached egg.

Calories: 107, **Protein:** 10 g, **Fat:** 6 g, **Carbohydrates:** 4 g, **Cholesterol:** 216 mg, **Fiber:** 0 g, **Sodium:** 877 mg

Cold Shrimp Soup

This is another one of those quick and easy soups that tastes like you spent hours cooking it. And, because it's pureed, you can buy the smallest, least expensive shrimp and no one can tell the difference.

2 cups low-fat buttermilk
1½ teaspoons dry mustard
¼ packet artificial sweetener
½ pound cooked shrimp, peeled and
　　cleaned
1 small cucumber, peeled, seeded, and
　　chopped (about ½ cup)
1 tablespoon minced fresh chives
Salt and pepper to taste

1.　In a food processor, combine all ingredients, except salt and pepper, and puree until smooth.
2.　Chill for 1 hour in refrigerator before serving. Add salt and pepper to taste.

Makes 4 servings

SERVING GUIDELINES

► **FOR GASTRIC SLEEVE AND BYPASS:**
　　Week 1: Liquid diet.
　　Weeks 2+: Serve ½–1 cup soup as is.

► **FOR BPD-DS:**
　　Week 1: Liquid diet.
　　Weeks 2+: Serve ½–1 cup soup as is.

► **FOR LAP-BAND:**
　　Week 1: Liquid diet.
　　Weeks 2+: Serve ½–1 cup soup as is.

► **FOR OTHERS:**
　　Serve 1 cup soup as is.

Calories: 90, **Protein:** 12 g, **Fat:** 2 g, **Carbohydrates:** 8 g, **Cholesterol:** 68 mg, **Fiber:** 0 g, **Sodium:** 410 mg

Creamy Shrimp Chowder

As you read down the list of ingredients for this recipe, you may be surprised by the cauliflower. Trust me, it works! It thickens like potato (which is in most chowders) without adding a lot of carbs. Note: Pureed, this soup tastes like the most outrageous shrimp bisque.

1 cup coarsely chopped cauliflower
Butter-flavored cooking spray
¼ cup chopped onion
1 teaspoon chopped garlic
1 ounce low-fat ham, finely diced
¼ teaspoon lemon-pepper
1 (8-ounce) bottle clam juice
1 cup evaporated fat-free milk
½ pound large shrimp, shelled and
    deveined, quartered
Salt and pepper to taste

1. Pour 2 cups water into a large saucepan. Place cauliflower in steamer insert, put into saucepan, cover, and steam over medium heat for 20 minutes, or until very soft.
2. Coat bottom of a large saucepan with cooking spray and cook onion and garlic over medium heat until soft, about 2 minutes.
3. Stir in ham and lemon-pepper, then add clam juice and evaporated milk.
4. Cook, stirring constantly, over medium heat until just barely boiling. Lower heat to low and simmer, stirring occasionally, for 10 minutes (it should be slightly thickened).
5. Puree ½ cauliflower and add to soup, stir well, and simmer for 5 minutes.
6. Coarsely chop remaining cauliflower and add to soup.
7. Stir in shrimp and cook for 30 seconds to 1 minute, or until all shrimp pieces turn pink.

Makes 4 servings

SERVING GUIDELINES

► **FOR GASTRIC SLEEVE AND BYPASS:**
  Week 1: Liquid diet.
  Weeks 2–3: Puree ½ cup soup.
  Weeks 4–7: Put ½ cup soup in mini-chopper and process until shrimp is chopped.
  Weeks 8+: Serve ½–1 cup soup as is.

► **FOR BPD-DS:**
  Week 1: Liquid diet.
  Weeks 2–3: Puree ½ cup soup.
  Weeks 4–7: Put ½ cup soup in mini-chopper and process until shrimp is chopped.
  Weeks 8+: Serve ½–1 cup soup as is.

► **FOR LAP-BAND:**
  Week 1: Liquid diet.
  Weeks 2–3: Puree ½ cup soup.
  Weeks 4–7: Put ½ cup soup in mini-chopper and process until shrimp is chopped.
  Weeks 8+: Serve ½–1 cup soup as is.

► **FOR OTHERS:**
  Serve 1 cup as is.

Calories: 130, **Protein:** 22 g, **Fat:** 2 g, **Carbohydrates:** 11 g, **Cholesterol:** 92 mg, **Fiber:** 1 g, **Sodium:** 647 mg

Mock Manhattan Clam Chowder

Chowder traditionally contains chunks of potatoes, but once you taste this chowder, you won't miss them. I use either chopped fresh clams from my local fish market or frozen chopped clams—never canned.

Olive oil cooking spray
1 cup chopped onion
3 large garlic cloves, minced
1 (28-ounce) can stewed tomatoes
½ pound cooked chopped fresh clams
2 tablespoons fresh basil, or 2
   teaspoons dried
⅛ teaspoon hot sauce (optional)
Salt and pepper to taste

1. Coat bottom of large nonstick saucepan with cooking spray and cook onion and garlic over low heat, covered, for 5 minutes, or until just translucent.
2. Add tomatoes, clams, basil, and hot sauce (if using), cover pan, and simmer for 5 minutes, or until heated through. Add salt and pepper to taste.

Makes 4 servings

► **Cooking Tip:** Instead of simmering on the stovetop, you can heat in the microwave—pour into glass bowl covered with plastic wrap and microwave on HIGH for 4 minutes.

SERVING GUIDELINES

► **FOR GASTRIC SLEEVE AND BYPASS:**
   Week 1: Liquid diet.
   Weeks 2–3: Puree ½ cup soup.
   Weeks 4+: Serve ½–1 cup soup as is.

► **FOR BPD-DS:**
   Week 1: Liquid diet.
   Weeks 2–3: Puree ½ cup soup.
   Weeks 4+: Serve ½–1 cup soup as is.

► **FOR LAP-BAND:**
   Week 1: Liquid diet.
   Weeks 2–3: Puree ½ cup soup.
   Weeks 4+: Serve ½–1 cup soup as is.

► **FOR OTHERS:**
   Serve 1 cup soup as is.

Calories: 117, **Protein:** 10 g, **Fat:** 1 g, **Carbohydrates:** 17 g, **Cholesterol:** 19 mg, **Fiber:** 4 g, **Sodium:** 60 mg

Mussel Bisque

This is one of those elegant creamy soups that tastes extravagantly rich, but it's not. Once you can start eating solid food, try making it without pureeing. You can serve this dish hot or cold.

Olive oil cooking spray
3 garlic cloves, minced
2 large shallots, minced
1 tablespoon fresh tarragon, or
   1½ teaspoons dried
¾ cup dry white wine
2 pounds (about 40) mussels,
   scrubbed and debearded
1 (8-ounce) bottle clam juice
¾ cup fat-free sour cream
Salt and pepper to taste

1. In a large stockpot, heat cooking spray over medium heat. Add garlic and shallots and cook, stirring, for 2 minutes, or until soft and translucent.
2. Add tarragon and cook for 30 seconds more. Remove shallot-garlic mixture from pot and put it aside.
3. Add wine to pot, bring to a boil, add mussels, and steam, covered, for 5 minutes, or until mussels open.
4. With a slotted spoon, remove mussels and let cool slightly.
5. Add clam juice and reserved shallot-garlic mixture back to liquid in pot and simmer, covered, for 10 minutes.
6. Remove cooled mussels from shell and place all mussel meat, soup, and sour cream in a food processor. Puree until smooth. Add salt and pepper to taste.

Makes 4 servings

SERVING GUIDELINES

➤ **FOR GASTRIC SLEEVE AND BYPASS:**
   Week 1: Liquid diet.
   Weeks 2+: Serve ½–1 cup soup as is.

➤ **FOR BPD-DS:**
   Week 1: Liquid diet.
   Weeks 2+: Serve ½–1 cup soup as is.

➤ **FOR LAP-BAND:**
   Week 1: Liquid diet.
   Weeks 2+: Serve ½–1 cup soup as is.

➤ **FOR OTHERS:**
   Serve 1 cup soup as is.

Calories: 234, **Protein:** 23 g, **Fat:** 4 g, **Carbohydrates:** 18 g, **Cholesterol:** 52 mg, **Fiber:** 0 g, **Sodium:** 572 mg

Mussels Posillipo

Sometimes called Zuppa di Mussels, this traditional southern Italian soup/main dish is a deliciously garlicky way to prepare this versatile shellfish. You can also substitute clams or shrimp.

Olive oil cooking spray
6 large garlic cloves, minced
2 tablespoons tomato paste
1 (28-ounce) can tomato puree
½ cup chopped fresh basil
2 teaspoons dried oregano
½ cup bottled clam juice
½ cup dry red wine
3 pounds mussels (about 60 mussels),
    cleaned and de-bearded
Salt and pepper to taste

1. In a large nonstick Dutch oven or stockpot, heat cooking spray over medium heat until hot but not smoking. Sauté garlic until soft, add tomato paste, and cook, stirring, until tomato paste browns.
2. Stir in tomato puree, basil, and oregano, lower heat, and cook, covered, for about 5 minutes.
3. Add clam juice and wine and bring to a boil. Cook, uncovered, for 5 minutes.
4. Add mussels and cover pot. Cook for 5 to 7 minutes, or until mussels open. Add salt and pepper to taste.

Makes 4 servings

SERVING GUIDELINES

➤ **FOR GASTRIC SLEEVE AND BYPASS:**
  Week 1: Liquid diet.
  Weeks 2–4: Puree 6 cooked mussels with ¼ cup vegetables and broth.
  Weeks 5–8: Chop 6 cooked mussels, and serve with ¼ cup vegetables and broth.
  Weeks 9+: Serve 6–12 cooked mussels with ¼–½ cup vegetables and broth.

➤ **FOR BPD-DS:**
  Week 1: Liquid diet.
  Weeks 2–3: Puree 6 cooked mussels with ¼ cup vegetables and broth.
  Weeks 4+: Serve 6–12 cooked mussels with ½–1 cup vegetables and broth.

➤ **FOR LAP-BAND:**
  Week 1: Liquid diet.
  Weeks 2–4: Puree 6 cooked mussels with ¼ cup vegetables and broth.
  Weeks 5–8: Chop 6 cooked mussels, serve with ¼ cup vegetables and broth.
  Weeks 9+: Serve 6–12 cooked mussels with ¼–½ cup vegetables and broth.

➤ **FOR OTHERS:**
  Serve 15 cooked mussels with 1 cup vegetables and broth.

Calories: 327, **Protein:** 33 g, **Fat:** 6 g, **Carbohydrates:** 32 g, **Cholesterol:** 67 mg, **Fiber:** 5 g, **Sodium:** 799 mg

Southwestern Tomato Soup

Here's a hearty soup with a real Tex-Mex kick. If you like it even spicier, don't be afraid to add more chili powder.

Olive oil cooking spray
½ cup finely chopped onion
2 tablespoons minced garlic
½ teaspoon chili powder
½ teaspoon ground cumin
½ teaspoon dried oregano
1 bay leaf
1 (14.5-ounce) can diced tomatoes
   with liquid
1 (14.5-ounce) can fat-free, low-sodium
   chicken broth
½ pound boneless, skinless turkey thighs
   (or any dark-meat turkey), cut up
Salt and pepper to taste

1. Coat bottom of a large soup pot with cooking spray. Over medium heat, sauté onion and garlic for 3 minutes.
2. Stir in chili powder, cumin, oregano, and bay leaf. Add tomatoes, chicken broth, and turkey, and bring to a boil.
3. Lower heat, cover, and simmer for 45 minutes. Remove bay leaf.
4. Puree in batches in a blender or food processor. Or you can use an immersion blender and puree right in soup pot. Add salt and pepper to taste.

Makes 4 servings

SERVING GUIDELINES

► **FOR GASTRIC SLEEVE AND BYPASS:**
   Week 1: Liquid diet.
   Weeks 2+ Serve ½–1 cup soup as is.

► **FOR BPD-DS:**
   Week 1: Liquid diet.
   Weeks 2+ Serve ½–1 cup soup as is.

► **FOR LAP-BAND:**
   Week 1: Liquid diet.
   Weeks 2+ Serve ½–1 cup soup as is.

► **FOR OTHERS:**
   Serve 1 cup as is.

Calories: 123, **Protein:** 14 g, **Fat:** 3 g, **Carbohydrates:** 9 g, **Cholesterol:** 39 mg, **Fiber:** 2 g, **Sodium:** 359 mg

Chilled Tomato Soup with Basil

This is a delectable, refreshing soup that has a sophisticated summer appeal. You can also serve it hot.

1 (28-ounce) can whole, peeled tomatoes
1 cup plain, fat-free yogurt
1 teaspoon ground cumin
2 teaspoons Worcestershire sauce
1½ cups fresh basil leaves

1. Puree tomatoes in a food processor until smooth.
2. Using a fine-mesh strainer, strain tomato puree over bowl, pressing solids to get as much liquid as possible. Then, discard seeds and solids left in strainer.
3. Pour strained tomato puree back into food processor, add yogurt, cumin, Worcestershire sauce, and 1 cup of basil leaves, and puree until smooth.
4. For garnish, finely mince remaining ½ cup of basil and sprinkle on top of individual servings.

Makes 4 servings

SERVING GUIDELINES

► **FOR GASTRIC SLEEVE AND BYPASS:**
 Week 1: Liquid diet.
 Weeks 2+: Serve ½–1 cup soup as is.

► **FOR BPD-DS:**
 Week 1: Liquid diet.
 Weeks 2+: Serve ½–1 cup soup as is.

► **FOR LAP-BAND:**
 Week 1: Liquid diet.
 Weeks 2+: Serve ½–1 cup soup as is.

► **FOR OTHERS:**
 Serve 1 cup soup as is.

Calories: 94, **Protein:** 7 g, **Fat:** 1 g, **Carbohydrates:** 16 g, **Cholesterol:** 1 mg, **Fiber:** 5 g, **Sodium:** 440 mg

Vegetables—Not Just an Aside

Vegetables that work with a meal or as a meal

WE'VE ALL HEARD the admonition to "eat your vegetables." But after weight reduction surgery, this can be a problem, as some people have trouble digesting certain vegetables in the weeks after surgery. So, in most of the recipe guidelines for this section, you'll notice that these dishes are not recommended for the first three to five weeks.

Of course, food tolerances can be very different for each person—for example, if you're like me, you'll be able to eat anything without any digestive sensitivity. If you're worried about adding vegetables back to your diet, try steaming and pureeing a small amount of various plain vegetables and see how you react. If it causes bloating or gas, don't try it again for at least two weeks to a month.

Okay, all caveats aside, let me tell you about these incredible vegetable recipes. They really put to rest the idea that vegetables are boring. We've used a variety of vegetables—mostly fresh, but we use a couple of frozen veggies in one or two recipes. You'll be amazed at the many different ways we've created to cook them—from simple purees to rich gratins, gutsy casseroles to delicate little pancakes, and even spicy chili and curry.

And here's where our ingenuity really paid off. We know that many people love mashed potatoes. But soft, buttery mashed potatoes are a real no-no when it comes to carbs and calories. When you cook cauliflower until soft, then puree it in your food processor with some rich-tasting reduced fat sour cream, it is sure to please any potato lover.

A lot of our veggie recipes (I think there are two exceptions) include protein from low-fat or fat-free cheeses, egg or egg white substitute, and soy nuts, which means they can be much more than just side dishes. You can eat them as delicious vegetarian main dishes for lunch or dinner. Some are even terrific for breakfast or brunch—such as Crustless Spinach and Cheese Quiche (page 47) or Zucchini Flan with Quick Tomato Sauce (page 53). Just be sure to check the protein levels to make sure that you're getting the amount you need every day. (Because some don't have as much protein, make sure you're not filling up on those alone.)

So, go ahead and "eat your vegetables" as soon as you can. They really make any eating program more varied, not to mention better balanced.

Note: The nutritional analyses are based on an average portion size (*Others'* portions).

Broccoli and Cheddar Gratin

I love pairing vegetables with cheese, and the addition of soy nuts gives this dish a bit of unexpected crunch (not to mention an extra measure of protein).

4 cups broccoli florets
Butter-flavored cooking spray
2 large garlic cloves, minced
¼ teaspoon crushed red pepper flakes
¼ cup low-fat, low-sodium vegetable broth
½ pound low-fat Cheddar cheese, grated
¼ cup ground soy nuts

1. Preheat oven to 400°F.
2. In a lidded pot fitted with a steamer basket, steam broccoli over ¾ cup water, covered, for 15 minutes, or until soft.
3. Coat a large skillet with cooking spray and sauté garlic and red pepper flakes over medium heat for 1 minute, or until just fragrant. Remove from heat and stir in broccoli, broth, and ¼ cup grated cheese.
4. Coat a 2-quart casserole with cooking spray and pour in broccoli-cheese mixture. Top with remaining cheese and sprinkle with ground soy nuts. Then, spray top with cooking spray.
5. Bake for about 12 minutes, or until cheese is melted and topping is golden.

Makes 4 servings

SERVING GUIDELINES

► **FOR GASTRIC SLEEVE AND BYPASS:**
Week 1: Liquid diet.
Weeks 2–4: Not recommended.
Weeks 5+: Serve ¼–½ cup cooked broccoli mixture as is.

► **FOR BPD-DS:**
Week 1: Liquid diet.
Weeks 2–4: Not recommended.
Weeks 5+: Serve ¼–½ cup cooked broccoli mixture as is.

► **FOR LAP-BAND:**
Week 1: Liquid diet.
Weeks 2–4: Not recommended.
Weeks 5+: Serve ¼–½ cup cooked broccoli mixture as is.

► **FOR OTHERS:**
Serve 1 cup cooked broccoli mixture as is.

Calories: 172, **Protein:** 20 g, **Fat:** 7 g, **Carbohydrates:** 9 g, **Cholesterol:** 12 mg, **Fiber:** 2 g, **Sodium:** 429 mg

Broccoli Soufflé

A soufflé is an elegant dish, but remember, once you take it out of the oven, serve it immediately or else it will collapse. (Don't worry—even if it collapses, it'll be just as delicious.)

1 (10-ounce) package frozen chopped broccoli, thawed and drained
Butter-flavored cooking spray
1 cup finely chopped onion
2 garlic cloves, minced
½ teaspoon hot sauce
1 cup skim evaporated milk
½ cup egg substitute
¼ cup grated Parmesan cheese
6 tablespoons egg white substitute
¼ teaspoon cream of tartar
Salt and pepper to taste

1. Preheat oven to 400°F.
2. Place broccoli in a double layer of paper towels and squeeze dry.
3. In a medium skillet, heat cooking spray over medium-high heat, add onion and garlic, and cook until onion is soft, about 5 minutes. Lower heat and add hot sauce and milk. Simmer for 4 minutes, stirring occasionally.
4. Place egg substitute in a small bowl and gradually add ½ cup of hot milk–onion mixture, stirring constantly with a whisk.
5. Add egg mixture back to skillet and cook over medium-low heat for 1 minute. Then, stir in broccoli and 3 tablespoons of cheese. Remove from heat and let cool.
6. In a medium bowl, beat egg white substitute and cream of tartar with an electric mixer until stiff peaks form.
7. Gently fold ¼ egg whites into broccoli mixture; then, fold in remaining egg whites.
8. Coat a 1½-quart soufflé dish with cooking spray. Spoon broccoli mixture into dish and sprinkle with remaining cheese.
9. Place dish in oven, lower temperature to 375°F, and bake for 40 minutes, or until puffy and set. Serve immediately. Add salt and pepper to taste.

Makes 4 servings

SERVING GUIDELINES

► **FOR GASTRIC SLEEVE AND BYPASS:**
   Week 1: Liquid diet.
   Weeks 2–4: Not recommended.
   Weeks 5+: Serve ¼–½ cup broccoli soufflé as is.

► **FOR BPD-DS:**
   Week 1: Liquid diet.
   Weeks 2–4: Not recommended.
   Weeks 5+: Serve ¼–½ cup broccoli soufflé as is.

► **FOR LAP-BAND:**
   Week 1: Liquid diet.
   Weeks 2–4: Not recommended.
   Weeks 5+: Serve ¼–½ cup broccoli soufflé as is.

► **FOR OTHERS:**
   Serve 1 cup broccoli soufflé as is.

Calories: 135, **Protein:** 14 g, **Fat:** 2 g, **Carbohydrates:** 17 g, **Cholesterol:** 4 mg, **Fiber:** 3 g, **Sodium:** 292 mg

Garlicky Broccoli and Ricotta

This is a great Italian peasant dish—rich, filling, and in our version, low fat. It also tastes good at room temperature.

1 bunch broccoli, trimmed and separated into large spears
Cooking spray
2 large garlic cloves, minced
1 cup fat-free ricotta cheese
1 teaspoon grated fresh ginger
¼ teaspoon red pepper flakes

1. In a lidded pot fitted with a steamer basket, steam broccoli over ¾ cup water, covered, until soft, 10 to 15 minutes.
2. Coat a small nonstick skillet with cooking spray and sauté garlic over medium heat until barely golden.
3. Cut broccoli into 1-inch pieces. Place broccoli, ricotta, garlic, and seasonings in a food processor and pulse until combined.

Makes 4 servings

SERVING GUIDELINES

► **FOR GASTRIC SLEEVE AND BYPASS:**
   Week 1: Liquid diet.
   Weeks 2–4: Not recommended.
   Weeks 5+: Serve ¼–½ cup cooked broccoli-ricotta mixture as is.

► **FOR BPD-DS:**
   Week 1: Liquid diet.
   Weeks 2–4: Not recommended.
   Weeks 5+: Serve ¼–½ cup cooked broccoli-ricotta mixture as is.

► **FOR LAP-BAND:**
   Week 1: Liquid diet.
   Weeks 2–4: Not recommended.
   Weeks 5+: Serve ¼–½ cup cooked broccoli-ricotta mixture as is.

► **FOR OTHERS:**
   Serve 1 cup cooked broccoli-ricotta mixture as is.

Calories: 88, **Protein:** 13 g, **Fat:** 1 g, **Carbohydrates:** 13 g, **Cholesterol:** 6 mg, **Fiber:** 5 g, **Sodium:** 71 mg

Garbanzo Guacamole

Sure, guacamole is a great party dip, but add garbanzo beans for protein and it's a terrific idea for lunch. Eat as is or use as a dip for raw veggies.

1 large garlic clove

⅔ cup canned low-sodium garbanzo beans (chickpeas), drained and rinsed

1 tablespoon fresh lemon juice

½ teaspoon ground cumin

1 medium avocado, peeled, pitted, and chopped (about ½ cup)

1 tablespoon chopped green chile

¾ cup canned low-sodium diced plum tomatoes, drained

½ cup finely chopped green onion (scallion)

Salt and pepper to taste

1. Place garlic clove in food processor and chop finely.
2. Add garbanzo beans, lemon juice, cumin, avocado, and chile, and puree until smooth.
3. Put bean-avocado mixture into a bowl and fold in tomatoes and green onion. Add salt and pepper to taste. Serve immediately.

Makes 2½ to 3 cups

SERVING GUIDELINES

▶ **FOR GASTRIC SLEEVE AND BYPASS:**
  Week 1: Liquid diet.
  Weeks 2+: Serve 2–3 ounces guacamole.

▶ **FOR BPD-DS:**
  Week 1: Liquid diet.
  Weeks 2+: Serve 2–3 ounces guacamole.

▶ **FOR LAP-BAND:**
  Week 1: Liquid diet.
  Weeks 2+: Serve 2–3 ounces guacamole.

▶ **FOR OTHERS:**
  Serve 4 ounces guacamole.

Calories: 115, **Protein:** 4 g, **Fat:** 5 g, **Carbohydrates:** 15 g, **Cholesterol:** 0 mg, **Fiber:** 5 g, **Sodium:** 97 mg

Cauliflower, Mushroom, and Cheddar Casserole

To me, this is one of those quintessential winter dishes—soft, pale, and rich with flavor. Of course, I spiffed it up a bit with roasted garlic and the crunch of a soy nut topping.

3 cups cauliflower florets, steamed until soft, about 12 minutes
1 cup chopped fresh white mushrooms
5 garlic cloves, roasted
½ pound low-fat Cheddar cheese, diced
Butter-flavored cooking spray
2 tablespoons ground soy nuts

1. Preheat oven to 350°F.
2. In a large bowl, mix together cauliflower, mushrooms, roasted garlic, and cheese.
3. Coat a small (8 x 8-inch) nonstick baking dish with cooking spray; pour in cauliflower mixture and sprinkle ground soy nuts on top.
4. Spray top with cooking spray and bake for 30 minutes.

Makes 4 servings

➤ **Cooking Tip:** To roast garlic, take whole unpeeled head of garlic and cut off top, or however many cloves you need. Drizzle with 1 teaspoon olive oil, wrap in foil, and bake at 275°F for 1½ to 2 hours. Can be stored in refrigerator for up to 1 week. Or you can roast garlic in the microwave: Cut the top off whole bulb of garlic, then place in a small glass bowl with ¼ cup chicken or vegetable broth and 1 teaspoon of olive oil. Cover tightly with plastic wrap and microwave on HIGH for 10 minutes. Let cool and peel.

SERVING GUIDELINES

➤ **FOR GASTRIC SLEEVE AND BYPASS:**
Week 1: Liquid diet.
Weeks 2–4: Not recommended.
Weeks 5+: Serve ¼–½ cup casserole as is.

➤ **FOR BPD-DS:**
Week 1: Liquid diet.
Weeks 2–4: Not recommended.
Weeks 5+: Serve ½–1 cup casserole as is.

➤ **FOR LAP-BAND:**
Week 1: Liquid diet.
Weeks 2–4: Not recommended.
Weeks 5+: Serve ¼–½ cup casserole as is.

➤ **FOR OTHERS:**
Serve 1 cup casserole as is.

Calories: 152, **Protein:** 18 g, **Fat:** 6 g, **Carbohydrates:** 9 g, **Cholesterol:** 12 mg, **Fiber:** 3 g, **Sodium:** 370 mg

Mashed Cauliflower

Okay, so it's not mashed potatoes, but it is delicious—smooth and soft and buttery-tasting, without all the calories and carbs.

3 cups cauliflower florets
⅔ cup skim milk
¼ cup fat-free sour cream
Salt and pepper to taste
20 sprays (5 per person) artificial
refrigerated butter spray (I Can't
Believe It's Not Butter works well)

1. Place cauliflower in a steamer insert in a 4-quart pot, cover, and steam over ¾ cup water for 10 to 15 minutes, or until very soft.
2. Place cooked cauliflower florets in a food processor and puree.
3. Add milk, sour cream, and salt and pepper to taste and puree until smooth.
4. Transfer mixture to microwave-safe dish and heat on HIGH for 2 minutes, then spray with butter spray.

Makes 4 servings

SERVING GUIDELINES

► **FOR GASTRIC SLEEVE AND BYPASS:**
 Week 1: Liquid diet.
 Weeks 2–4: Not recommended.
 Weeks 5+: Serve ¼–½ cup mashed cauliflower
 as is.

► **FOR BPD-DS:**
 Week 1: Liquid diet.
 Weeks 2–4: Not recommended.
 Weeks 5+: Serve ½–1 cup mashed cauliflower
 as is.

► **FOR LAP-BAND:**
 Week 1: Liquid diet.
 Weeks 2–4: Not recommended.
 Weeks 5+: Serve ¼–½ cup mashed cauliflower
 as is.

► **FOR OTHERS:**
 Serve 1 cup mashed cauliflower as is.

Calories: 202, **Protein:** 16 g, **Fat:** 1 g, **Carbohydrates:** 36 g, **Cholesterol:** 13 mg, **Fiber:** 8 g, **Sodium:** 225 mg

Creamed Spinach

At last, a low-fat version of everyone's favorite side dish. It tastes as rich and creamy as the original.

1 (10-ounce) package frozen chopped spinach, thawed
Butter-flavored cooking spray
¼ cup thinly sliced shallots
⅓ cup skim milk
½ cup fat-free cream cheese
¼ teaspoon ground nutmeg (optional)
Salt and pepper to taste

1. Place thawed spinach in two layers of paper towels and squeeze to remove as much liquid as possible.
2. Coat a saucepan with cooking spray and heat over medium heat until hot.
3. Add shallots and sauté until lightly browned.
4. Lower heat, add milk, cream cheese, and nutmeg (if using), and whisk until smooth.
5. Stir in spinach, cover pan, and simmer for 10 minutes. Remove lid, increase heat to medium, and cook for 1 minute more to thicken slightly. Add salt and pepper to taste.

Makes 4 servings

SERVING GUIDELINES

➤ **FOR GASTRIC SLEEVE AND BYPASS:**
Week 1: Liquid diet.
Weeks 2–4: Not recommended.
Weeks 5+: Serve ¼–½ cup creamed spinach as is.

➤ **FOR BPD-DS:**
Week 1: Liquid diet.
Weeks 2–4: Not recommended.
Weeks 5+: Serve ½–1 cup creamed spinach as is.

➤ **FOR LAP-BAND:**
Week 1: Liquid diet.
Weeks 2–4: Not recommended.
Weeks 5+: Serve ¼–½ cup creamed spinach as is.

➤ **FOR OTHERS:**
Serve 1 cup creamed spinach as is.

Calories: 62, **Protein:** 7 g, **Fat:** 0 g, **Carbohydrates:** 7 g, **Cholesterol:** 5 mg, **Fiber:** 3 g, **Sodium:** 206 mg

Crustless Spinach and Cheese Quiche

This is, without a doubt, one of my favorite vegetable dishes. It's a basic quiche—custard and cheese—that you don't always have to make with spinach (sometimes I use broccoli, asparagus, or zucchini, and I've even been known to add diced red bell pepper). So, go ahead, experiment—but remember, the nutritional numbers may change.

Butter-flavored cooking spray
¾ cup chopped fresh white mushrooms
¼ cup chopped shallots
2 (10-ounce) packages frozen chopped spinach
1 tablespoon water
¼ cup egg substitute
½ cup skim milk
½ cup diced low-fat Swiss cheese
¼ teaspoon ground nutmeg

1. Spray a microwaveable casserole dish with cooking spray. Add mushrooms and shallots, cover dish, and microwave on HIGH for 1 minute.
2. Place frozen spinach and water on top of mushroom mixture. Cover and microwave on HIGH for 3½ minutes.
3. Uncover and break up spinach, flipping it over. Re-cover and microwave on HIGH for another 3½ minutes. Remove from microwave and drain if too liquidy.
4. In a separate bowl, combine egg substitute and milk and stir in diced cheese and nutmeg.
5. Stir spinach-mushroom-shallot mixture in casserole dish to combine. Pour egg-milk-cheese mixture on top, cover, and microwave on HIGH for 4 minutes.

Makes 4 servings

SERVING GUIDELINES

► **FOR GASTRIC SLEEVE AND BYPASS:**
  Week 1: Liquid diet.
  Weeks 2–4: Not recommended.
  Weeks 5+: Serve ¼–½ cup quiche as is.

► **FOR BPD-DS:**
  Week 1: Liquid diet.
  Weeks 2–4: Not recommended.
  Weeks 5+: Serve ½–1 cup quiche as is.

► **FOR LAP-BAND:**
  Week 1: Liquid diet.
  Weeks 2–4: Not recommended.
  Weeks 5+: Serve ¼–½ cup quiche as is.

► **FOR OTHERS:**
  Serve 1 cup quiche as is.

Calories: 143, **Protein:** 16 g, **Fat:** 4 g, **Carbohydrates:** 10 g, **Cholesterol:** 16 mg, **Fiber:** 5 g, **Sodium:** 221 mg

Kale with Apple and Onion

Unlike most of the other vegetable dishes in this book, this one has no protein, so it really is only a side dish. I love to serve it with most of the pork recipes we've created. We adapted this recipe from *Gourmet* magazine.

1 medium Granny Smith apple, peeled and cored
Olive oil cooking spray
¾ cup chopped onion
⅛ teaspoon curry powder
1 bunch kale, tough stems and ribs removed, coarsely chopped (about 4 cups)
½ cup water

1. Cut apple into wedges, then into ¼-inch slices.
2. Coat a 4- to 5-quart nonstick pot with cooking spray and heat over medium-high heat until hot but not smoking. Sauté onion, stirring occasionally, until golden.
3. Stir in apple and curry powder, lower heat, cover pot, and cook for 2 minutes, or until apple is almost tender.
4. Add kale and water and cook, covered, for about 5 minutes, or until kale is tender and most of liquid has evaporated.

Makes 4 servings

► **Cooking tip:** To make this a main dish, try browning a pound of ground pork or turkey until almost crisp, about 15 minutes, then mix it into the kale-apple-onion mixture. *This will change the nutritional analysis.*

SERVING GUIDELINES

► **FOR GASTRIC SLEEVE AND BYPASS:**
Week 1: Liquid diet.
Weeks 2–4: Not recommended.
Weeks 5+: Serve ¼–½ cup cooked kale-apple-onion as is.

► **FOR BPD-DS:**
Week 1: Liquid diet.
Weeks 2–4: Not recommended.
Weeks 5+: Serve ½–1 cup cooked kale-apple-onion as is.

► **FOR LAP-BAND:**
Week 1: Liquid diet.
Weeks 2–4: Not recommended.
Weeks 5+: Serve ¼–½ cup cooked kale-apple-onion as is.

► **FOR OTHERS:**
Serve 1 cup cooked kale-apple-onion as is.

Calories: 66, **Protein:** 3 g, **Fat:** 1 g, **Carbohydrates:** 15 g, **Cholesterol:** 0 mg, **Fiber:** 3 g, **Sodium:** 30 mg

Marinated String Beans

Another purely side dish vegetable recipe (no protein). I always think of this recipe as perfect summer food—great on a picnic. You can serve it hot alongside beef or lamb, or serve it cold as a substitute for coleslaw.

½ pound string beans, tips cut off
2 cups diced seeded tomato
5 garlic cloves, peeled and cut in half horizontally
1 tablespoon dried basil
¼ cup water
2 teaspoons olive oil
1 tablespoon balsamic vinegar
Salt and freshly ground pepper to taste

1. In a medium microwave-safe bowl, combine beans, tomato, garlic, basil, and water.
2. Cover and microwave on HIGH for 9 minutes, or until beans are soft.
3. Let bean mixture cool and then toss with oil, vinegar, and salt and pepper to taste.
4. Serve it hot or cold (if you don't like a strong garlic flavor, remove garlic before serving).

Makes 4 servings

SERVING GUIDELINES

▶ **FOR GASTRIC SLEEVE AND BYPASS:**
Week 1: Liquid diet.
Weeks 2–4: Not recommended.
Weeks 5+: Serve ¼–½ cup marinated beans as is.

▶ **FOR BPD-DS:**
Week 1: Liquid diet.
Weeks 2–4: Not recommended.
Weeks 5+: Serve ½–1 cup marinated beans as is.

▶ **FOR LAP-BAND:**
Week 1: Liquid diet.
Weeks 2–4: Not recommended.
Weeks 5+: Serve ¼–½ cup marinated beans as is.

▶ **FOR OTHERS:**
Serve 1 cup marinated beans as is.

Calories: 58, **Protein:** 2 g, **Fat:** 3 g, **Carbohydrates:** 8 g, **Cholesterol:** 0 mg, **Fiber:** 2 g, **Sodium:** 249 mg

Minted Cucumbers with Yogurt

You'll find a version of this recipe in Indian cooking as well as in Middle Eastern and Greek cuisines. It's very refreshing, especially when served with spicy dishes. Use it in a chunky state as a side dish, or puree it and serve as a sauce over fish or grilled lamb.

2 large cucumbers, peeled and seeded
  (about 3 cups)
1 cup plain, fat-free yogurt
1 garlic clove, peeled and quartered
2 teaspoons fresh lemon juice
½ teaspoon ground cumin
2 teaspoons minced fresh mint leaves, or
  1 teaspoon dried

1. Dice cucumbers.
2. Combine all ingredients, except cucumbers, in a food processor and process until smooth.
3. In a large bowl, toss cucumbers with yogurt mixture.

Makes 4 servings

SERVING GUIDELINES

► **FOR GASTRIC SLEEVE AND BYPASS:**
  Week 1: Liquid diet.
  Weeks 2–4: Not recommended.
  Weeks 5+: Serve ¼–½ cup cucumber-yogurt mixture as is.

► **FOR BPD-DS:**
  Week 1: Liquid diet.
  Weeks 2–4: Not recommended.
  Weeks 5+: Serve ½–1 cup cucumber-yogurt mixture as is.

► **FOR LAP-BAND:**
  Week 1: Liquid diet.
  Weeks 2–4: Not recommended.
  Weeks 5+: Serve ¼–½ cup cucumber-yogurt mixture as is.

► **FOR OTHERS:**
  Serve 1 cup cucumber-yogurt mixture as is.

Calories: 68, **Protein:** 5 g, **Fat:** 0 g, **Carbohydrates:** 12 g, **Cholesterol:** 2 mg, **Fiber:** 2 g, **Sodium:** 69 mg

Pattypan Squash Puree

If you've never tried these delicate little veggies, you've missed out. This puree is as elegant as anything you'll find in fine restaurants, and it's really fun to watch friends and family guess what's in it.

1 pound green baby pattypan squash, halved and stemmed

2 shallots, peeled and cut in half (about ¼ cup)

½ cup fat-free sour cream

½ cup fat-free cream cheese

1 tablespoon prepared horseradish

½ teaspoon dried thyme

Salt and pepper to taste

1. Place squash and shallots in a steamer basket in a saucepan, cover, and steam over ¾ cup water over medium heat for 15 minutes, or until soft.
2. Remove squash and shallots from pan and place in a food processor. Add sour cream, cream cheese, horseradish, and thyme and process until smooth. Add salt and pepper to taste.

Makes 4 servings

SERVING GUIDELINES

► **FOR GASTRIC SLEEVE AND BYPASS:**
Week 1: Liquid diet.
Weeks 2–4: Not recommended.
Weeks 5+: Serve ¼–½ cup cooked squash puree as is.

► **FOR BPD-DS:**
Week 1: Liquid diet.
Weeks 2–4: Not recommended.
Weeks 5+: Serve ½–1 cup cooked squash puree as is.

► **FOR LAP-BAND:**
Week 1: Liquid diet.
Weeks 2–4: Not recommended.
Weeks 5+: Serve ¼–½ cup cooked squash puree as is.

► **FOR OTHERS:**
Serve ½–1 cup squash puree as is.

Calories: 103, **Protein:** 8 g, **Fat:** 1 g, **Carbohydrates:** 16 g, **Cholesterol:** 10 mg, **Fiber:** 2 g, **Sodium:** 211 mg

Zucchini and Ricotta Rustica

The Italians have a delicious dish called Torta Rustica, a pie filled with cheeses, vegetables, and fresh herbs. We've taken it out of the piecrust and added some Canadian bacon for a slightly smoky flavor.

Olive oil cooking spray
2 medium zucchini, thinly sliced (about 3 cups)
½ pound Canadian bacon, sliced thin, trimmed of fat and diced
1½ cups diced fresh tomato
½ cup shredded fresh basil
½ cup fat-free ricotta cheese
2 tablespoons grated Parmesan cheese
Salt and pepper to taste

1. In a large nonstick skillet, heat cooking spray until hot but not smoking. Add zucchini, and sauté over medium heat until softened.
2. Stir in Canadian bacon, tomato, and basil and cook until tomato is softened.
3. Remove from heat and toss with ricotta and Parmesan cheeses.
4. Add salt and pepper to taste.

Makes 4 servings

SERVING GUIDELINES

► **FOR GASTRIC SLEEVE AND BYPASS:**
  Week 1: Liquid diet.
  Weeks 2–4: Not recommended.
  Weeks 5+: Serve ¼–½ cup cooked zucchini mixture as is.

► **FOR BPD-DS:**
  Week 1: Liquid diet.
  Weeks 2–4: Not recommended.
  Weeks 5+: Serve ½–1 cup cooked zucchini mixture as is.

► **FOR LAP-BAND:**
  Week 1: Liquid diet.
  Weeks 2–4: Not recommended.
  Weeks 5+: Serve ¼–½ cup cooked zucchini mixture as is.

► **FOR OTHERS:**
  Serve ½–1 cup cooked zucchini mixture as is.

Calories: 150, **Protein:** 19 g, **Fat:** 5 g, **Carbohydrates:** 9 g, **Cholesterol:** 5 mg, **Fiber:** 2 g, **Sodium:** 702 mg

Zucchini Flan with Quick Tomato Sauce

A perfect recipe for weekend brunch or a light dinner. You'll probably have some tomato sauce left over—I save it to use on chicken or fish. You can even freeze the leftover sauce in ice cube trays to defrost and use later.

Flan:

Olive oil cooking spray
4 cups thinly sliced zucchini
1 tablespoon minced garlic
½ cup thinly sliced onion
1 cup egg substitute
¼ cup skim milk

**Quick Tomato Sauce
(makes approximately 1½ cups):**

Olive oil cooking spray
1 garlic clove, minced
1 (14.5-ounce) can diced tomatoes
2 tablespoons chopped fresh basil leaves
1 packet artificial sweetener
   (Splenda or Truvia)
Salt and pepper to taste

1. Preheat oven to 350°F.
2. *To make flan:* Coat a large nonstick skillet with cooking spray, add zucchini, and sauté over medium heat for about 10 minutes, stirring occasionally, until zucchini wilts and gives up its liquid.
3. Add garlic and onion and continue to cook until zucchini browns slightly. Turn off heat and let cool.
4. In a large bowl, beat together egg substitute and milk. Add zucchini mixture to eggs.
5. Coat an 8½ x 4½-inch loaf pan with cooking spray and pour zucchini-egg mixture into it.
6. Place loaf pan in a large baking dish and pour hot water around loaf pan until baking dish is as full as possible without getting water into loaf pan. Bake until flan is set but still wobbly in middle, about 30 minutes. Remove from oven and cool on rack for about 5 minutes.
7. *While flan is baking, make sauce:* Coat a small saucepan with cooking spray and brown garlic for 1 minute. Stir in tomatoes, basil, and sweetener and simmer for 5 to 7 minutes.
8. Invert loaf pan over a plate and unmold flan, then slice. Serve with tomato sauce on side.

Makes 4 servings

SERVING GUIDELINES

- **FOR GASTRIC SLEEVE AND BYPASS:**
  Week 1: Liquid diet.
  Weeks 2–4: Puree ¼–½ cup flan with 2
    tablespoons sauce until smooth.
  Weeks 5+: Serve ¼–½ cup flan topped with 2
    tablespoons sauce.

- **FOR BPD-DS:**
  Week 1: Liquid diet.
  Weeks 2–3: Puree ¼–½ cup flan with 2
    tablespoons sauce until smooth.
  Weeks 4+: Serve ½–1 cup flan topped with 2
    tablespoons sauce.

- **FOR LAP-BAND:**
  Week 1: Liquid diet.
  Weeks 2–4: Puree ¼–½ cup flan with 2
    tablespoons sauce until smooth.
  Weeks 5+: Serve ¼–½ cup flan topped with 2
    tablespoons sauce.

- **FOR OTHERS:**
  Serve 1 cup flan with 2 tablespoons sauce.

Zucchini Flan:

Calories: 71, **Protein:** 9 g, **Fat:** 0 g, **Carbohydrates:** 9 g, **Cholesterol:** 0 mg, **Fiber:** 2 g, **Sodium:** 114 mg

Quick Tomato Sauce (2 tablespoons):

Calories: 9, **Protein:** 0 g, **Fat:** 0 g, **Carbohydrates:** 2 g, **Cholesterol:** 0 mg, **Fiber:** 0 g, **Sodium:** 39 mg

Zucchini Custards

These are dainty little custards that look simply lovely on a plate—almost as delicate as a soufflé, but extremely flavorful. I usually serve them with lamb or fish.

3 cups grated zucchini
Cooking spray
¼ cup minced shallots
½ cup egg substitute
3 tablespoons egg white substitute
¾ cup skim milk
1½ tablespoons dried basil
1 teaspoon dried oregano
¼ teaspoon ground nutmeg
⅛ teaspoon ground cayenne pepper
3 tablespoons grated Parmesan cheese

1. Preheat oven to 350°F.
2. Spread grated zucchini on two layers of paper towels, cover with additional paper towels, and let stand 15 minutes, pressing occasionally until barely moist.
3. Coat bottom of a small nonstick skillet with cooking spray and sauté shallots over medium-high heat until lightly browned, about 6 minutes.
4. In bowl of your food processor, combine egg substitute, egg white substitute, milk, and seasonings and process until well blended.
5. Add zucchini, cheese, and shallots and pulse until combined.
6. Coat eight small (4-ounce) ramekins with cooking spray and spoon zucchini mixture into cups. Place ramekins in a baking pan and pour about 1 inch of hot water into pan, being careful not to spill any water into ramekins. Bake for 40 minutes.
7. Serve in ramekins or run knife around inside edges of ramekins and invert onto plates.

Makes 8 servings

SERVING GUIDELINES

- **FOR GASTRIC SLEEVE AND BYPASS:**
  Week 1: Liquid diet.
  Weeks 2+: Serve 1 custard as is.

- **FOR BDP-DS:**
  Week 1: Liquid diet.
  Weeks 2+: Serve 1 custard as is.

- **FOR LAP-BAND:**
  Week 1: Liquid diet.
  Weeks 2+: Serve 1 custard as is.

- **FOR OTHERS:**
  Serve 1 custard as is.

Calories: 38, **Protein:** 4 g, **Fat:** 1 g, **Carbohydrates:** 4 g, **Cholesterol:** 2 mg, **Fiber:** 1 g, **Sodium:** 84 mg

Zucchini Pancakes

These are such fun—light and delicate, fresh and green. You can serve them at breakfast, brunch, lunch, or dinner. They're especially good as a side dish with fish.

4 cups grated zucchini
    (from about 1 pound)
¼ cup grated Parmesan cheese
¼ cup chopped fresh basil
2 tablespoons chopped fresh chives
1 packet artificial sweetener
    (Splenda or Truvia)
6 tablespoons egg white substitute
Olive oil cooking spray
½ cup fat-free sour cream
Salt and pepper to taste

1. Place grated zucchini in a colander, let stand for 20 minutes at room temperature, then wrap zucchini in three layers of paper towels, top with another three layers of towels, and wring out as much liquid as possible.
2. Place zucchini in a bowl and mix with cheese, basil, chives, and sweetener.
3. In a separate bowl, beat egg whites with an electric mixer until they hold stiff peaks, then gently fold into zucchini mixture.
4. Heat cooking spray in a 10-inch nonstick skillet over moderately high heat until hot but not smoking. Spoon 2 tablespoons of zucchini mixture per pancake into skillet (skillet should accommodate about 5 pancakes at a time), flattening slightly, and sauté for 3 minutes each side, turning once, until golden brown.
5. Transfer cooked pancakes to plate and keep warm. Re-spray skillet and repeat cooking steps until all remaining batter is cooked.
6. Top with fat-free sour cream and add salt and pepper to taste.

Makes 4 servings (16 pancakes)

SERVING GUIDELINES

► **FOR GASTRIC SLEEVE AND BYPASS:**
    Week 1: Liquid diet.
    Weeks 2–4: Not recommended.
    Weeks 5+: Serve 1–2 pancakes with 2
        tablespoons sour cream.

► **FOR BPD-DS:**
    Week 1: Liquid diet.
    Weeks 2–4: Not recommended.
    Weeks 5+: Serve 2–4 pancakes with 2
        tablespoons sour cream.

► **FOR LAP-BAND:**
    Week 1: Liquid diet.
    Weeks 2–4: Not recommended.
    Weeks 5+: Serve 1–2 pancakes with 2
        tablespoons sour cream.

► **FOR OTHERS:**
    Serve 4 pancakes with 2 tablespoons sour cream.

Calories: 89, **Protein:** 8 g, **Fat:** 2 g, **Carbohydrates:** 11 g, **Cholesterol:** 9 mg, **Fiber:** 2 g, **Sodium:** 161 mg

Main Course

Meat, poultry, seafood, and vegetarian entrées to please your palate

THIS IS REALLY the meat (pardon the pun) of any cookbook. We've created recipes that give you an incredible variety of flavors, textures, ethnic influences, and cooking styles. That's because Michele and I know that there's nothing more boring than an eating program that depends on one small group of ingredients or just relegates you to broiling and baking your food.

Every recipe has been developed to taste great in whatever form you're eating it—pureed, chopped, or as cooked. You'll find elegant quick sautés and succulent slow-cooked stews. There are spicy marinated dishes and taste bud–tingling curries. There's an exotic *tagine* from Morocco as well as a tropical seafood salad from the Caribbean. You can even make Italian-style lasagna, using our two luscious pasta-free recipes. And, of course, we've included a number of delectably simple American dishes.

Every recipe is protein rich, low fat, and has no "bad" carbohydrates. We use lean cuts of meat, skinless poultry, and lots of different fish and shellfish, plus tofu, beans, and low-fat or fat-free cheeses.

There are a lot of cooking tricks out there involving ingredients and techniques that can be used to make sure you don't feel deprived, but it takes time and experimentation to figure them out. You don't have to do it—we did it for you. For instance, once you're past your soft-food period, we teach you how to add crunch to a dish by topping it with chopped nuts or ground soy nuts—a great source of protein. We'll even show you how to use them to bread cutlets that are "fried" using cooking spray.

Of course, the greatest reward after having weight reduction surgery is achieving your weight-loss goals. But along the way, this cookbook will make each meal a reward in itself.

Note: The nutritional analyses are based on an average portion size (*Others'* portions).

Deviled Chicken Spread

Need an idea for lunch, a great appetizer, or maybe something to bring to a party? This spread is great on crackers, with raw veggies or mixed with hard-boiled egg yolks to make special deviled eggs.

1 cup cubed cooked chicken breast
½ cup low-fat mayonnaise
2 tablespoons Dijon mustard
⅓ cup coarsely chopped sweet onion
2 tablespoons paprika
1 teaspoon lemon-pepper
½ teaspoon chili powder, or to taste

1. In bowl of a food processor, combine chicken and mayonnaise and puree until smooth.
2. Add all other ingredients and puree until very smooth.

Makes 4 servings

SERVING GUIDELINES

▶ **FOR GASTRIC SLEEVE AND BYPASS:**
  Week 1: Liquid diet.
  Weeks 2+: Serve 2–3 ounces deviled chicken.

▶ **FOR BPD-DS:**
  Week 1: Liquid diet.
  Weeks 2+: Serve 2–3 ounces deviled chicken.

▶ **FOR LAP-BAND:**
  Week 1: Liquid diet.
  Weeks 2+: Serve 2–3 ounces deviled chicken.

▶ **FOR OTHERS:**
  Serve 4 ounces deviled chicken.

Calories: 104, **Protein:** 12 g, **Fat:** 3 g, **Carbohydrates:** 8 g, **Cholesterol:** 25 mg, **Fiber:** 1 g, **Sodium:** 592 mg

BBQ-Baked Chicken

This is for people who like really tangy barbecue sauce. This chicken also tastes great served cold.

Marinade:
½ cup apple cider
¼ cup tomato paste
Brown-sugar artificial sweetener
  (1 teaspoon equivalent)
1 tablespoon cider vinegar
1 teaspoon dried thyme
½ teaspoon Asian chili paste with garlic

1 pound skinless, boneless chicken thighs
Canola oil cooking spray

1. Preheat oven to 350°F.
2. *To make marinade:* In a small bowl, combine all marinade ingredients and stir well.
3. Reserve ¼ cup and place remaining marinade and chicken in large resealable plastic bag. Shake to coat, then refrigerate for 1 hour.
4. Remove chicken from bag and place in a nonstick baking pan that has been coated with cooking spray.
5. Bake chicken for 45 minutes, or until juices run clear when pierced with a fork. Remove chicken from pan and keep warm.
6. Skim any fat from pan juices and discard. Pour skimmed pan juices into a small saucepan and add reserved ¼ cup marinade. Stir over low heat for 2 minutes. Pour over chicken.

Makes 4 servings

SERVING GUIDELINES

▸ **FOR GASTRIC SLEEVE AND BYPASS:**
  Week 1: Liquid diet.
  Weeks 2–4: Puree 2 ounces cooked chicken with 2 tablespoons sauce.
  Weeks 5–7: Chop 2 ounces cooked chicken and top with sauce.
  Weeks 8+: Serve 2–4 ounces cooked chicken topped with sauce.

▸ **FOR BPD-DS:**
  Week 1: Liquid diet.
  Weeks 2–3: Puree 3–4 ounces cooked chicken with 2 tablespoons sauce.
  Weeks 4+: Serve 3–4 ounces cooked chicken topped with sauce.

▸ **FOR LAP-BAND:**
  Week 1: Liquid diet.
  Weeks 2–4: Puree 2 ounces cooked chicken with 2 tablespoons sauce.
  Weeks 5–7: Chop 2 ounces cooked chicken and top with sauce.
  Weeks 8+: Serve 2–4 ounces cooked chicken topped with sauce.

▸ **FOR OTHERS:**
  Serve 4 ounces cooked chicken topped with sauce.

Calories: 164, **Protein:** 24 g, **Fat:** 5 g, **Carbohydrates:** 7 g, **Cholesterol:** 94 mg, **Fiber:** 1 g, **Sodium:** 118 mg

Chicken and Fresh Apricot Tagine

This is one of the most delectable chicken recipes I know, and according to people who have spent time in the Middle East, very authentic. You can substitute water-packed canned apricots, but I prefer to wait until fresh ones are in season.

Canola oil cooking spray
Salt and pepper to taste
1 pound skinless, boneless chicken thighs
1 pound skinless, boneless chicken breast,
    quartered
2 cups thinly sliced yellow onion
1 large garlic clove, minced
1½ pounds (10–12) small ripe apricots,
    quartered and pitted
1½ teaspoons ground cinnamon
¼ teaspoon ground ginger
¼ teaspoon ground coriander
¼ teaspoon saffron threads
⅔ cup fat-free, low-sodium chicken broth
6 packets artificial sweetener
    (Splenda or Truvia)

1. In a pot large enough to hold all chicken pieces in one layer, heat cooking spray over medium-high heat until hot but not smoking.
2. Salt and pepper chicken and brown in pot for about 4 minutes on each side. Transfer chicken to a paper towel–lined plate.
3. Add onion to pot and cook, stirring occasionally, for 5 minutes, or until lightly browned.
4. Add garlic and sauté for 1 minute. Stir in apricots, cinnamon, ginger, coriander, saffron, broth, and sweetener.
5. Place chicken on top of apricot mixture and cover. Lower heat to low and cook for 45 to 50 minutes, or until chicken is cooked through and sauce is thickened.
6. If sauce has not thickened at end of cooking time, transfer chicken to preheated 200°F oven to keep warm. Reduce sauce, uncovered, over medium heat until thick.

Makes 8 servings

SERVING GUIDELINES

► **FOR GASTRIC SLEEVE AND BYPASS:**
   Week 1: Liquid diet.
   Weeks 2–4: Puree 2 ounces cooked chicken with 2 tablespoons apricot sauce.
   Weeks 5–7: Chop 2 ounces cooked chicken and top with apricot sauce.
   Weeks 8+: Serve 2–4 ounces cooked chicken topped with apricot sauce.

► **FOR BPD-DS:**
   Week 1: Liquid diet.
   Weeks 2–3: Puree 2–3 ounces cooked chicken with 2 tablespoons apricot sauce.
   Weeks 4+: Serve 3–4 ounces cooked chicken topped with apricot sauce.

► **FOR LAP-BAND:**
   Week 1: Liquid diet.
   Weeks 2–4: Puree 2 ounces cooked chicken with 2 tablespoons apricot sauce.
   Weeks 5–7: Chop 2 ounces cooked chicken and top with apricot sauce.
   Weeks 8+: Serve 2–4 ounces cooked chicken topped with apricot sauce.

► **FOR OTHERS:**
   Serve 4 ounces cooked chicken topped with apricot sauce.

Calories: 297, **Protein:** 29 g, **Fat:** 4 g, **Carbohydrates:** 40 g, **Cholesterol:** 80 mg, **Fiber:** 9 g, **Sodium:** 147 mg

Walnut-Crusted Chicken Bits with Deviled Raspberry-Apple Dipping Sauce

This is fun food. Great for a party, an appetizer or a "small plates" meal. You can make the chicken and sauce a day ahead and serve them at room temperature.

Chicken Bits:

2 cups fat-free buttermilk

1 teaspoon garlic powder

½ teaspoon lemon-pepper

1 teaspoon ground allspice

1 pound skinless boneless chicken breast, cut into 1½-inch cubes

½ cup egg white substitute, or whites of 3 large eggs

¾ cup finely chopped walnuts

Canola oil cooking spray

Raspberry-Apple Dipping Sauce:

1 (8-ounce) jar unsweetened applesauce

3 tablespoons seedless sugar-free raspberry or grape preserves

2 tablespoons Dijon mustard

1. *To make chicken:* In a large bowl, combine buttermilk, garlic powder, lemon-pepper, and allspice. Place chicken in a large resealable plastic bag. Add buttermilk mixture, close bag, and toss until well coated, then refrigerate for at least 1 hour (you can marinate in refrigerator up to 1 day ahead).
2. Preheat oven to 400°F and line a baking sheet with aluminum foil.
3. Drain chicken in a large colander.
4. In a large bowl, lightly beat egg whites. Toss chicken pieces with egg whites.
5. Roll chicken pieces in chopped walnuts to coat.
6. Spray foil-covered baking sheet with cooking spray and spread chicken pieces in an even layer on sheet.
7. Bake chicken for 15 to 20 minutes, or until cooked through.
8. *While chicken is baking, make sauce:* Place all sauce ingredients in a medium bowl and mix until well combined. Serve chicken with sauce on the side.

Serves 6 to 8 people as an appetizer

SERVING GUIDELINES

- **FOR GASTRIC SLEEVE AND BYPASS:**
  Week 1: Liquid diet.
  Weeks 2–4: Puree 2 ounces cooked chicken with 2 tablespoons sauce.
  Weeks 5–7: Chop 2 ounces cooked chicken, serve with 2 tablespoons sauce.
  Weeks 8+: Serve 2–4 ounces cooked chicken with 2 tablespoons sauce.

- **FOR BPD-DS:**
  Week 1: Liquid diet.
  Weeks 2–4: Puree 2 ounces cooked chicken with 2 tablespoons sauce.
  Weeks 5–7: Chop 2 ounces cooked chicken, serve with 2 tablespoons sauce.
  Weeks 8+: Serve 2–4 ounces cooked chicken with 2 tablespoons sauce.

- **FOR LAP-BAND:**
  Week 1: Liquid diet.
  Weeks 2–4: Puree 2 ounces cooked chicken with 2 tablespoons sauce.
  Weeks 5–7: Chop 2 ounces cooked chicken, serve with 2 tablespoons sauce.
  Weeks 8+: Serve 2–4 ounces cooked chicken with 2 tablespoons sauce.

- **FOR OTHERS:**
  Serve 4 ounces cooked chicken with sauce.

Calories: 365, **Protein:** 37 g, **Fat:** 16 g, **Carbohydrates:** 21 g, **Cholesterol:** 57 mg, **Fiber:** 5 g, **Sodium:** 725 mg

Chicken and Spinach Adobo

This is an adaptation of a classic Filipino recipe. It's got a little bit of a kick from the red pepper, which some people like to kick higher by adding more.

¼ cup cider vinegar
¼ cup light soy sauce
1 garlic clove, minced
1 bay leaf
¼ teaspoon red pepper flakes
1 pound boneless, skinless chicken thighs
Canola cooking spray
1 (10-ounce) package chopped frozen
　spinach, thawed

1. In a bowl, mix together vinegar, soy sauce, garlic, bay leaf, and red pepper flakes.
2. Pour into a large resealable plastic bag, add chicken, and turn bag to coat. Marinate in refrigerator for 2 hours, turning occasionally. Remove chicken from bag and reserve marinade.
3. Coat a large nonstick lidded skillet with cooking spray and sauté chicken over medium-high heat for 7 minutes, turning to brown evenly.
4. While chicken is browning, place spinach in two layers of paper towels and squeeze out moisture.
5. Remove chicken from pan. Then, pour reserved marinade into pan and bring to a boil.
6. Stir in spinach and place chicken on top. Lower heat, cover pan, and cook for 10 minutes.
7. Remove chicken from pan and keep warm. Increase heat to medium-high and reduce liquid by half, 5 to 7 minutes.

Makes 4 servings

SERVING GUIDELINES

▶ **FOR GASTRIC SLEEVE AND BYPASS:**
　Week 1: Liquid diet.
　Weeks 2–4: Puree 2 ounces cooked chicken with 2 tablespoons spinach and sauce.
　Weeks 5–7: Chop 2 ounces cooked chicken and top with spinach and sauce.
　Weeks 8+: Serve 2–4 ounces cooked chicken topped with spinach and sauce.

▶ **FOR BPD-DS:**
　Week 1: Liquid diet.
　Weeks 2–3: Puree 3–4 ounces cooked chicken with 2 tablespoons spinach and sauce.
　Weeks 4+: Serve 3–4 ounces cooked chicken topped with spinach and sauce.

▶ **FOR LAP-BAND:**
　Week 1: Liquid diet.
　Weeks 2–4: Puree 2 ounces cooked chicken with 2 tablespoons spinach and sauce.
　Weeks 5–7: Chop 2 ounces cooked chicken and top with spinach and sauce.
　Weeks 8+: Serve 2–4 ounces cooked chicken topped with spinach and sauce.

▶ **FOR OTHERS:**
　Serve 4 ounces cooked chicken topped with spinach and sauce.

Calories: 169, **Protein:** 26 g, **Fat:** 5 g, **Carbohydrates:** 5 g, **Cholesterol:** 94 mg, **Fiber:** 3 g, **Sodium:** 694 mg

Spanish Chicken and "Rice"

Here is a perfect recipe for a weeknight: quick, easy, and absolutely delicious. I use frozen cauliflower rice so it's *almost* authentic. Feel free to make it with shrimp or tofu instead of chicken.

Olive oil cooking spray
1 pound boneless, skinless chicken breast, cut into 1-inch pieces
1 medium onion, diced
2 garlic cloves, minced
1 large green bell pepper, seeded and diced
1 large red, yellow, or orange bell pepper, seeded and diced
2 tablespoons tomato paste
¼ cup low-sodium chicken broth
1 (14.5 ounce) can low-sodium diced tomatoes; drained, reserving ¼ cup liquid
1 teaspoon ground cumin
½ teaspoon lemon-pepper
1 teaspoon sweet or smoked paprika
1 (12-ounce) bag frozen cauliflower rice

1. In a deep lidded skillet, heat cooking spray over medium-high heat until hot but not smoking.
2. When it starts to shimmer, add chicken pieces and stir until barely cooked through, 5 to 7 minutes.
3. Transfer chicken to a plate, then re-spray pan. Add onion, garlic, and diced peppers and cook, stirring, until vegetables are soft, 3 to 5 minutes.
4. Stir in tomato paste, and cook, stirring, until it begins to darken, 2 to 3 minutes. Pour in broth, tomatoes, reserved tomato liquid, and spices and stir well.
5. Add frozen cauliflower rice, breaking up any lumps, stir, and cover. Cook, stirring occasionally, for 8 to 10 minutes, then add chicken back to skillet.
6. If it looks too soupy, increase heat to high and cook for another 2 to 3 minutes until dry.

Makes 4 servings

SERVING GUIDELINES

➤ **FOR GASTRIC SLEEVE AND BYPASS:**
 Week 1: Liquid diet.
 Week 2–7: Puree 2 ounces cooked chicken and cauliflower rice.
 Weeks 8+: Serve 2–4 ounces cooked chicken with cauliflower rice.

➤ **FOR BPD-DS:**
 Week 1: Liquid diet.
 Week 2–7: Puree 2 ounces cooked chicken and cauliflower rice.
 Weeks 8+: Serve 2–4 ounces cooked chicken with cauliflower rice.

➤ **FOR LAP-BAND:**
 Week 1: Liquid diet.
 Week 2–7: Puree 2 ounces cooked chicken and cauliflower rice.
 Weeks 8+: Serve 2–4 ounces cooked chicken with cauliflower rice.

➤ **FOR OTHERS:**
 Serve 4 ounces cooked chicken with cauliflower rice.

Calories: 194, **Protein:** 26 g, **Fat:** 3 g, **Carbohydrates:** 14 g, **Cholesterol:** 55 mg, **Fiber:** 5 g, **Sodium:** 749 mg

Chicken Beau Séjour

This sophisticated recipe is usually made with veal. One day I had the brilliant idea to try it with chicken and have made it that way ever since. The vinegar and thyme are a classic French flavor combination.

Canola oil cooking spray
1 pound boneless, skinless chicken breast
2 teaspoons fresh thyme leaves, or 1 teaspoon dried
2 bay leaves
4 large garlic cloves, sliced in half horizontally
½ pound white mushrooms, thickly sliced
2 tablespoons red wine vinegar
½ cup fat-free, low-sodium chicken broth
Salt and pepper to taste

1. In a large nonstick lidded skillet, heat cooking spray over medium-high heat. Add chicken, brown on one side, then turn.
2. Sprinkle chicken with thyme and place one bay leaf on each piece. Arrange garlic, cut side down, around chicken and layer mushroom slices over garlic. Cover pan and cook over low heat for 15 minutes.
3. Remove chicken and mushrooms from pan and keep warm. Discard bay leaves.
4. Deglaze pan with vinegar and bring to a simmer, scraping up any browned bits. Add chicken broth to pan, press down on garlic to mash (if you don't want so pungent a garlic flavor, remove and discard garlic before adding broth).
5. Simmer broth for 2 minutes until slightly reduced. Add back to skillet chicken and mushrooms and any chicken juices that have accumulated. Add salt and pepper to taste.

Makes 4 servings

SERVING GUIDELINES

► **FOR GASTRIC SLEEVE AND BYPASS:**
  Week 1: Liquid diet.
  Weeks 2–4: Puree 2 ounces cooked chicken with 2 tablespoons mushroom sauce until smooth.
  Weeks 5–7: Chop 2 ounces cooked chicken and top with mushroom sauce.
  Weeks 8+: Serve 2–4 ounces cooked chicken with mushroom sauce.

► **FOR BPD-DS:**
  Week 1: Liquid diet.
  Weeks 2–3: Puree 2–3 ounces cooked chicken with 2 tablespoons mushroom sauce until smooth.
  Weeks 4+: Serve 3–4 ounces cooked chicken with mushroom sauce.

► **FOR LAP-BAND:**
  Week 1: Liquid diet.
  Weeks 2–4: Puree 2 ounces cooked chicken with 2 tablespoons sauce until smooth.
  Weeks 5–7: Chop 2 ounces cooked chicken and top with mushroom sauce.
  Weeks 8+: Serve 2–4 ounces cooked chicken with mushroom sauce.

► **FOR OTHERS:**
  Serve 4 ounces cooked chicken with mushroom sauce.

Calories: 147, **Protein:** 28 g, **Fat:** 2 g, **Carbohydrates:** 4 g, **Cholesterol:** 66 mg, **Fiber:** 1 g, **Sodium:** 162 mg

Chicken Breasts Stuffed with Ham and Cheese

We've updated a classic, making it lighter and, we think, better. With just a white wine and mushroom sauce instead of a heavy cream sauce, you really taste how well all the flavors complement one another.

1 pound chicken breast cutlets, pounded very thinly
4 ounces lean boiled ham, sliced thinly (4 slices)
4 ounces low-fat Swiss cheese, sliced thinly (4 slices)
Cooking spray
1 cup thinly sliced fresh mushrooms
1 large shallot, finely minced
½ cup dry white wine
¼ cup fat-free, low-sodium chicken broth
1 teaspoon dried tarragon
Salt and pepper to taste

1. Cut pounded chicken into eight thin cutlets. Lay out four cutlets; top each with a slice of ham and a slice of cheese, and then top each with a second cutlet.
2. Coat a large nonstick skillet with cooking spray and sauté stuffed chicken cutlets over medium-high heat, carefully turning once, for 8 to 10 minutes, until golden and cooked through. Transfer to a plate and keep warm.
3. Re-spray pan and sauté mushrooms and shallot over medium-high heat, stirring, for 3 minutes. Add wine to deglaze pan, stirring to scrape up any browned bits, and simmer until it's reduced by half.
4. Add chicken broth and tarragon and simmer for 2 minutes. Stir in any chicken juices that have accumulated on plate and add salt and pepper to taste.

Makes 4 servings

SERVING GUIDELINES

- **FOR GASTRIC SLEEVE AND BYPASS:**
  Week 1: Liquid diet.
  Weeks 2–4: Puree 2 ounces cooked stuffed cutlets with 2 tablespoons sauce.
  Weeks 5–7: Chop 2 ounces cooked stuffed cutlets and top with sauce.
  Weeks 8+: Serve 2–4 ounces cooked stuffed cutlets topped with sauce.

- **FOR BPD-DS:**
  Week 1: Liquid diet.
  Weeks 2–3: Puree 2–3 ounces cooked stuffed cutlets with 2 tablespoons sauce.
  Weeks 4+: Serve 3–4 ounces cooked stuffed cutlets topped with sauce.

- **FOR LAP-BAND:**
  Week 1: Liquid diet.
  Weeks 2–4: Puree 2 ounces cooked stuffed cutlets with 2 tablespoons sauce.
  Weeks 5–7: Chop 2 ounces cooked stuffed cutlets and top with sauce.
  Weeks 8+: Serve 2–4 ounces cooked stuffed cutlets topped with sauce.

- **FOR OTHERS:**
  Serve 4 ounces cooked stuffed cutlets topped with sauce.

Calories: 266, **Protein:** 41 g, **Fat:** 6 g, **Carbohydrates:** 4 g, **Cholesterol:** 93 mg, **Fiber:** 0 g, **Sodium:** 435 mg

Chicken Breasts with Creamy Tomato Sauce

Too rich to be a tomato sauce and too light to be a cream sauce, this creamy tomato sauce is a great combination of flavors that tops off chicken cutlets deliciously.

Butter-flavored cooking spray
1 pound chicken breast cutlets
½ pound fresh mushrooms, quartered
1 large shallot, finely minced
¼ cup white wine
½ cup canned diced tomatoes, drained
½ cup evaporated fat-free milk
Salt and pepper to taste

1. Coat a large nonstick skillet with cooking spray and sauté chicken over medium-high heat for about 3 minutes per side, until golden and cooked through. Transfer chicken to a plate and keep warm.
2. Re-spray pan and sauté mushrooms and shallot over medium-high heat, stirring, for 3 minutes. Add wine to deglaze pan, stirring to scrape up any browned bits, until it's reduced by half. Add tomatoes and cook, stirring occasionally, for 3 to 4 minutes.
3. Lower heat to low and add evaporated milk. Cook, stirring constantly, for 6 to 8 minutes, or until reduced by half. Stir in any chicken juices that have accumulated on plate and add salt and pepper to taste.

Makes 4 servings

SERVING GUIDELINES

► **FOR GASTRIC SLEEVE AND BYPASS:**
  Week 1: Liquid diet.
  Weeks 2–4: Puree 2 ounces cooked chicken with 2 tablespoons sauce.
  Weeks 5–7: Chop 2 ounces cooked chicken and top with sauce.
  Weeks 8+: Serve 2–4 ounces cooked chicken topped with sauce.

► **FOR BPD-DS:**
  Week 1: Liquid diet.
  Weeks 2–3: Puree 2–3 ounces cooked chicken with 2 tablespoons sauce.
  Weeks 4+: Serve 3–4 ounces cooked chicken topped with sauce.

► **FOR LAP-BAND:**
  Week 1: Liquid diet.
  Weeks 2–4: Puree 2 ounces cooked chicken with 2 tablespoons sauce.
  Weeks 5–7: Chop 2 ounces cooked chicken and top with sauce.
  Weeks 8+: Serve 2–4 ounces cooked chicken topped with sauce.

► **FOR OTHERS:**
  Serve 4 ounces cooked chicken topped with sauce.

Calories: 188, **Protein:** 31 g, **Fat:** 2 g, **Carbohydrates:** 9 g, **Cholesterol:** 66 mg, **Fiber:** 1 g, **Sodium:** 165 mg

Chicken with Shallots and Tiny Tomatoes

I love those little grape tomatoes. I eat 'em like candy. Paired with rich, dark meat chicken thighs in a flavorful herbed mustard sauce, they turn a quick recipe into something special.

Olive oil cooking spray
4 skinless, boneless chicken thighs
12 medium shallots, peeled
1½ cups dry white cooking wine or low-sodium chicken broth
2 tablespoons Dijon mustard
1 teaspoon dried tarragon
2 cups halved grape tomatoes

1. Spray a large lidded skillet with cooking spray. Heat over medium-high heat until it shimmers.
2. Sauté chicken thighs, turning occasionally, until well browned on all sides, 5 to 7 minutes. Remove from pan.
3. Re-spray pan and cook shallots until they soften and begin to caramelize, 10 to 12 minutes. Stir in wine and scrape up any browned bits.
4. Stir in mustard and tarragon, then add chicken back to skillet. Cover skillet, lower heat to low, and cook for 15 minutes.
5. Uncover skillet and add tomatoes, then simmer for another 10 minutes, or until sauce is slightly thickened.

Makes 4 servings

SERVING GUIDELINES

▸ **FOR GASTRIC SLEEVE AND BYPASS:**
  Week 1: Liquid diet.
  Weeks 2–4: Puree 2 ounces cooked chicken and vegetables with 2 tablespoons sauce.
  Weeks 5–7: Chop 2 ounces cooked chicken and vegetables with 2 tablespoons sauce.
  Weeks 8+: Serve 2–4 ounces cooked chicken and vegetables with 2 tablespoons sauce.

▸ **FOR BPD-DS:**
  Week 1: Liquid diet.
  Weeks 2–3: Puree 2 ounces cooked chicken and vegetables with 2 tablespoons sauce.
  Weeks 4–8+: Serve 2–4 ounces cooked chicken and vegetables with 2 tablespoons sauce.

▸ **FOR LAP-BAND:**
  Week 1: Liquid diet.
  Weeks 2–4: Puree 2 ounces cooked chicken and vegetables with 2 tablespoons sauce.
  Weeks 5–7: Chop 2 ounces cooked chicken and vegetables with 2 tablespoons sauce.
  Weeks 8+: Serve 2–4 ounces cooked chicken and vegetables with 2 tablespoons sauce.

▸ **FOR OTHERS:**
  Serve 4 ounces cooked chicken and vegetables with sauce.

Calories: 377, **Protein:** 30 g, **Fat:** 10 g, **Carbohydrates:** 25 g, **Cholesterol:** 92 mg, **Fiber:** 7 g, **Sodium:** 580 mg

Chicken Sauté with Mushrooms

My mother used to tease me that I bought mushrooms the way most people bought bread and milk. This recipe really highlights the earthy taste of the mushrooms in a light creamy, tarragon-scented sauce.

Olive oil cooking spray
1 pound chicken breast cutlets
3 tablespoons minced shallots
2 cups sliced fresh mushrooms
½ cup white wine
¾ cup fat-free, low-sodium chicken broth
½ cup plain, fat-free yogurt
½ packet artificial sweetener
   (Splenda or Truvia)
1 tablespoon minced fresh tarragon
   leaves, or ½ teaspoon dried
Salt and pepper to taste

1. In a large nonstick skillet, heat cooking spray over medium-high heat until hot but not smoking. Sauté chicken for 3 minutes on each side until golden brown and no longer pink inside. Remove chicken from pan and keep warm.
2. Re-spray pan, add shallots and mushrooms, and cook, stirring, for about 2 minutes, or until tender. Pour in wine, increase heat to high, and cook for 2 minutes.
3. Add broth and cook for 3 to 5 minutes, or until reduced by half. Lower heat to low and stir in yogurt and sweetener. Cook for about 2 minutes, or until thick enough to coat spoon.
4. Stir in tarragon and season with salt and pepper to taste.

Makes 4 servings

SERVING GUIDELINES

▸ **FOR GASTRIC SLEEVE AND BYPASS:**
   Week 1: Liquid diet.
   Weeks 2–4: Puree 2 ounces cooked chicken with mushrooms and 2 tablespoons sauce.
   Weeks 5–7: Chop 2 ounces cooked chicken and top with mushrooms and sauce.
   Weeks 8+: Serve 2–4 ounces cooked chicken with mushrooms and sauce.

▸ **FOR BPD-DS:**
   Week 1: Liquid diet.
   Weeks 2–3: Puree 2 ounces cooked chicken with mushrooms and 2 tablespoons sauce.
   Weeks 4+: Serve 3–4 ounces cooked chicken topped with mushrooms and sauce.

▸ **FOR LAP-BAND:**
   Week 1: Liquid diet.
   Weeks 2–4: Puree 2 ounces cooked chicken with mushrooms and 2 tablespoons sauce.
   Weeks 5–7: Chop 2 ounces cooked chicken and top with mushrooms and sauce.
   Weeks 8+: Serve 2–4 ounces cooked chicken with mushrooms and sauce.

▸ **FOR OTHERS:**
   Serve 4 ounces cooked chicken with mushrooms and sauce.

Calories: 181, **Protein:** 30 g, **Fat:** 2 g, **Carbohydrates:** 6 g, **Cholesterol:** 66 mg, **Fiber:** 1 g, **Sodium:** 230 mg

Grilled Veggies with Quick-Marinated Chicken, Fish, or Steak

I love grilled vegetables so much, once the summer is over, I grill them under the broiler. They're so soft and flavorful that they almost make a luscious sauce with any kind of broiled protein.

Marinade:

⅓ cup light sodium soy sauce

½ cup fresh orange juice

½ teaspoon garlic powder

1 teaspoon grated fresh ginger, or ½ teaspoon ground ginger

¼ teaspoon chili powder

¼ teaspoon sesame oil

1 pound your choice of protein: boneless skinless chicken breast, thick fish fillet, or flank steak

Grilled Vegetables:

Olive oil cooking spray

2 medium sweet onions, thickly sliced

2 large tomatoes, thickly sliced

4 portobello mushroom caps

1 large red, yellow, or orange bell pepper, seeded and cut into 4 pieces

1 medium zucchini, quartered

2 teaspoons lemon-pepper

1. Preheat broiler and arrange rack to top position.
2. *To make marinade:* In a shallow baking dish, combine all marinade ingredients.
3. If using flank steak, use a sharp knife to make diagonal cuts about ¼ inch deep on surface of meat. Add your protein of choice to marinade, cover with foil or plastic wrap, and marinate at room temperature while vegetables are cooking.
4. *To grill vegetables:* Cover a large baking sheet with aluminum foil and spray with cooking spray.
5. Arrange all vegetables on baking sheet, spray with cooking spray, and sprinkle with lemon-pepper. Place baking sheet in oven on highest rack and broil for 30 minutes, or until nice and charred. Move baking sheet to lowest rack to keep veggies warm while you broil the protein.
6. Reserving marinade, remove protein from marinade and pat dry. Pour marinade into a small saucepan and bring to a simmer. Simmer over low heat for 8 to 10 minutes, or until slightly reduced.
7. *To broil protein:* Place chicken, fish, or steak in a lightly sprayed broiler pan and broil on top rack for 8 to 10 minutes, turning once. Remove from oven and test for doneness.
8. Remove vegetables from oven. Serve vegetables and protein together with reduced marinade.

Makes 4 servings

► **Note:** If you have any leftovers, they're just as good cold to take for lunch.

SERVING GUIDELINES

► **FOR GASTRIC SLEEVE AND BYPASS:**
Week 1: Liquid diet.
Weeks 2–7: Puree 2 ounces cooked protein with 2 tablespoons grilled veggies.
Weeks 8+: Serve 2–4 ounces cooked protein topped with 2 tablespoons grilled veggies.

► **FOR BPD-DS:**
Week 1: Liquid diet.
Weeks 2–7: Puree 2 ounces cooked protein with 2 tablespoons grilled veggies.
Weeks 8+: Serve 2–4 ounces cooked protein topped with 2 tablespoons grilled veggies.

► **FOR LAP-BAND:**
Week 1: Liquid diet.
Weeks 2–7: Puree 2 ounces cooked protein with 2 tablespoons grilled veggies.
Weeks 8+: Serve 2–4 ounces cooked protein topped with 2 tablespoons grilled veggies.

► **FOR OTHERS:**
Serve 4 ounces cooked protein topped with grilled veggies.

Calories: 225, **Protein:** 32 g, **Fat:** 2 g, **Carbohydrates:** 19 g, **Cholesterol:** 66 mg, **Fiber:** 4 g, **Sodium:** 1,173 mg

Middle Eastern Chicken

If you've ever tasted shawarma, you know it's a flavor bomb street food, often made with lamb. I use chicken and a lot less oil for a lighter version. It tastes great with Yogurt-Mint Sauce (page 196) or Tikka Yogurt Sauce (page 197).

Marinade:

⅓ cup fresh lemon juice
2 teaspoons olive oil
3 garlic cloves, peeled and minced
½ teaspoon kosher salt
1 teaspoon freshly ground black pepper
1 teaspoon ground cumin
1 teaspoon paprika
¼ teaspoon ground turmeric
¼ teaspoon ground cinnamon
1 teaspoon crushed red pepper flakes

4 to 6 skinless, boneless chicken thighs
Olive oil cooking spray
1 large red onion, peeled and quartered

1. *To make marinade:* In a large bowl, whisk to combine all marinade ingredients.
2. Add chicken and toss well to coat. Cover and store in refrigerator for at least 1 hour up to overnight.
3. When ready to cook, preheat oven to 425°F and spray a rimmed sheet pan with cooking spray.
4. Add onion to chicken and marinade in bowl, and toss once to combine.
5. Spread chicken and onion, well coated with marinade, on prepared sheet pan and roast until chicken is crisp and browned at edges and cooked through, 30 to 40 minutes.
6. Remove from oven, let rest for 2 minutes, then slice into small pieces.

Makes 4 servings

SERVING GUIDELINES

► **FOR GASTRIC SLEEVE AND BYPASS:**
Week 1: Liquid diet.
Weeks 2–4: Puree 2 ounces cooked chicken and onion with 2 tablespoons broth or stock.
Weeks 5–7: Chop 2 ounces cooked chicken and onion.
Weeks 8+: Serve 2–4 ounces cooked chicken and onion.

► **FOR BPD-DS:**
Week 1: Liquid diet.
Weeks 2–3: Puree 2 ounces cooked chicken and onion with 2 tablespoons broth or stock.
Weeks 4+: Serve 2–4 ounces cooked chicken and onion.

► **FOR LAP-BAND:**
Week 1: Liquid diet.
Weeks 2–4: Puree 2 ounces cooked chicken and onion with 2 tablespoons broth or stock.
Weeks 5–7: Chop 2 ounces cooked chicken and onion.
Weeks 8+: Serve 2–4 ounces cooked chicken and onion.

► **FOR OTHERS:**
Serve 4 ounces cooked chicken and onion.

Calories: 170, **Protein:** 23 g, **Fat:** 7 g, **Carbohydrates:** 5 g, **Cholesterol:** 105 mg, **Fiber:** 1 g, **Sodium:** 143 mg

Spicy Grilled Marinated Chicken Breasts

We were looking for a tasty grilled chicken recipe and Michele came up with this one. Not only do the citrus and spices make the chicken tangy, they actually make it mouth-meltingly tender. You can also make this dish in the broiler.

Marinade:

½ cup low-fat sour cream
1 tablespoon fresh lime juice
2 tablespoons fresh orange juice
1 tablespoon fresh lemon juice
1 tablespoon chili powder
1 tablespoon paprika
½ teaspoon cayenne pepper
⅛ teaspoon freshly ground black pepper
2 tablespoons chopped fresh tarragon
   leaves, or ½ teaspoon dried

1 pound chicken breasts
Canola cooking spray

1. *To make marinade:* Whisk marinade ingredients together and set aside.
2. Trim chicken of any fat and arrange in a shallow dish, just large enough to hold chicken in one layer. Add marinade and toss to coat. Marinate chicken, covered, for 6 to 24 hours in refrigerator.
3. Prepare grill.
4. Reserving marinade, remove chicken from marinade, letting excess drip off, and place marinade in a small saucepan.
5. Spray grill rack with cooking spray and grill chicken for about 5 minutes on each side or until cooked through.
6. Over medium-low heat, bring reserved marinade to a simmer. Simmer for 8 to 10 minutes; you should have about ½ cup. If needed, add up to ¼ cup chicken broth and 1 tablespoon low-fat sour cream for last 2 minutes, stirring gently. Spoon over cooked chicken.

Makes 4 servings

➤ **Variation:** If broiling, spray broiler pan with cooking spray, place chicken on pan, and broil on the top rack about 5 minutes on each side or until cooked through.

SERVING GUIDELINES

➤ **FOR GASTRIC SLEEVE AND BYPASS:**
   Week 1: Liquid diet.
   Weeks 2–4: Puree 2 ounces cooked chicken with 2 tablespoons reserved marinade.
   Weeks 5–7: Chop 2 ounces cooked chicken.
   Weeks 8+: Serve 2–4 ounces cooked chicken.

➤ **FOR BPD-DS:**
   Week 1: Liquid diet.
   Weeks 2–3: Puree 2 ounces cooked chicken with 2 tablespoons reserved marinade.
   Weeks 4+: Serve 3–4 ounces cooked chicken.

➤ **FOR LAP-BAND:**
   Week 1: Liquid diet.
   Weeks 2–4: Puree 2 ounces cooked chicken with 2 tablespoons reserved marinade.
   Weeks 5–7: Chop 2 ounces cooked chicken.
   Weeks 8+: Serve 2–4 ounces cooked chicken.

➤ **FOR OTHERS:**
   Serve 4 ounces cooked chicken.

Calories: 185, **Protein:** 30 g, **Fat:** 2 g, **Carbohydrates:** 11 g, **Cholesterol:** 71 mg, **Fiber:** 1 g, **Sodium:** 120 mg

Turkey Cutlets Francese

This has been one of my favorite recipes for years. By dipping the cutlets in egg and Parmesan, you don't miss the traditional breading at all.

½ cup grated Parmesan cheese
¼ cup dried parsley flakes
1 cup egg substitute
¼ cup skim milk
1 pound turkey cutlets, thinly sliced
Olive oil cooking spray
½ cup white wine
2 tablespoons concentrated chicken broth

1. On a flat plate, mix Parmesan cheese and parsley.
2. In a baking dish or platter with sides, mix eggs and milk. Dip cutlets into egg, then into cheese mixture, then back into egg.
3. Coat a nonstick skillet with cooking spray and heat over medium-high heat until hot but not smoking. Sauté cutlets for 3 minutes on each side, or until browned. Transfer to a plate and keep warm.
4. Lower heat to low, pour wine into pan, and simmer, stirring to scrape up any browned bits.
5. Add concentrated chicken broth and continue to simmer, stirring, for 2 more minutes, or until sauce reduces slightly.

Makes 4 servings

SERVING GUIDELINES

► **FOR GASTRIC SLEEVE AND BYPASS:**
Week 1: Liquid diet.
Weeks 2–4: Puree 2 ounces cooked cutlet with 2 tablespoons sauce.
Weeks 5–7: Chop 2 ounces cooked cutlet and top with 2 tablespoons sauce.
Weeks 8+: Serve 2–4 ounces cooked cutlet topped with 2 tablespoons sauce.

► **FOR BPD-DS:**
Week 1: Liquid diet.
Weeks 2–3: Puree 2 ounces cooked cutlet with 2 tablespoons sauce.
Weeks 4+: Serve 2–4 ounces cooked cutlet topped with 2 tablespoons sauce.

► **FOR LAP-BAND:**
Week 1: Liquid diet.
Weeks 2–4: Puree 2 ounces cooked cutlet with 2 tablespoons sauce.
Weeks 5–7: Chop 2 ounces cooked cutlet and top with 2 tablespoons sauce.
Weeks 8+: Serve 2–4 ounces cooked cutlet topped with 2 tablespoons sauce.

► **FOR OTHERS:**
Serve 4 ounces cooked cutlet topped with 2 tablespoons sauce.

Calories: 255, **Protein:** 38 g, **Fat:** 7 g, **Carbohydrates:** 7 g, **Cholesterol:** 76 mg, **Fiber:** 0 g, **Sodium:** 839 mg

Turkey Cacciatore

This dish is just like chicken cacciatore, only we happen to think it's better. Wait until you taste how the dark turkey meat stands up to the gutsy southern Italian flavors.

Olive oil cooking spray
1 pound skinless, boneless turkey thighs
   (or any dark turkey meat)
1 cup chopped onion
2 garlic cloves, minced
2 tablespoons sun-dried tomato paste
1 (14.5-ounce) can whole tomatoes
¼ cup chopped fresh basil
1 teaspoon dried oregano
¼ teaspoon red pepper flakes
½ cup dry red wine
Salt and pepper to taste

1. Heat cooking spray in a large nonstick pot over medium-high heat until hot but not smoking. Cook turkey for 3 minutes until browned all over and remove from pot.
2. Add onion and garlic and sauté for 2 minutes, or until lightly browned. Add tomato paste and cook, stirring, until paste starts to darken.
3. Put turkey back into pot, add all other ingredients, and stir well.
4. Cover, lower heat to low, and simmer for 30 minutes until turkey is tender.

Makes 4 servings

SERVING GUIDELINES

▶ **FOR GASTRIC SLEEVE AND BYPASS:**
   Week 1: Liquid diet.
   Weeks 2–4: Puree 2 ounces cooked turkey with 2 tablespoons sauce until smooth.
   Weeks 5–7: Chop 2 ounces cooked turkey and top with 2 tablespoons sauce.
   Weeks 8+: Serve 2–4 ounces cooked turkey topped with 2 tablespoons sauce.

▶ **FOR BPD-DS:**
   Week 1: Liquid diet.
   Weeks 2–3: Puree 2–3 ounces cooked turkey with 2 tablespoons sauce until smooth.
   Weeks 4+: Serve 2–4 ounces cooked turkey topped with 2 tablespoons sauce.

▶ **FOR LAP-BAND:**
   Week 1: Liquid diet.
   Weeks 2–4: Puree 2 ounces cooked turkey with 2 tablespoons sauce until smooth.
   Weeks 5–7: Chop 2 ounces cooked turkey and top with 2 tablespoons sauce.
   Weeks 8+: Serve 2–4 ounces cooked turkey topped with 2 tablespoons sauce.

▶ **FOR OTHERS:**
   Serve 4 ounces cooked turkey topped with 2 tablespoons sauce.

Calories: 224, **Protein:** 26 g, **Fat:** 5 g, **Carbohydrates:** 13 g, **Cholesterol:** 78 mg, **Fiber:** 3 g, **Sodium:** 256 mg

Turkey Paprikash

This is an updated, lighter version of a creamy, earthy Hungarian classic.

Butter-flavored cooking spray
1 pound boneless, skinless turkey thighs
   (or any dark turkey meat)
¼ cup chopped onion
1 garlic clove, minced
¼ pound (about 10) fresh mushrooms,
   sliced
1 tablespoon sweet paprika
1½ teaspoons tomato paste
¼ teaspoon cayenne pepper
¼ cup fat-free, low-sodium chicken broth
2 tablespoons fat-free sour cream
Salt to taste

1. Heat cooking spray in a medium skillet over medium-high heat until hot but not smoking. Sauté turkey for 2 minutes to brown on each side.
2. Add onion and garlic, cover, lower heat, and cook for 20 minutes, or until turkey is cooked through. Remove turkey from pan and keep warm.
3. Stir mushrooms, paprika, tomato paste, cayenne, and chicken broth into pan and cook, covered, for 3 minutes. Remove from heat and stir in sour cream and salt to taste.
4. Add turkey back to skillet and turn to coat.

Makes 4 servings

SERVING GUIDELINES

▶ **FOR GASTRIC SLEEVE AND BYPASS:**
   Week 1: Liquid diet.
   Weeks 2–4: Puree 2 ounces cooked turkey with 2 tablespoons sauce until smooth.
   Weeks 5–7: Chop 2 ounces cooked turkey and top with 2 tablespoons sauce.
   Weeks 8+: Serve 2–4 ounces cooked turkey topped with 2 tablespoons sauce.

▶ **FOR BPD-DS:**
   Week 1: Liquid diet.
   Weeks 2–3: Puree 2–3 ounces cooked turkey with 2 tablespoons sauce until smooth.
   Weeks 4+: Serve 2–4 ounces cooked turkey topped with 2 tablespoons sauce.

▶ **FOR LAP-BAND:**
   Week 1: Liquid diet.
   Weeks 2–4: Puree 2 ounces cooked turkey with 2 tablespoons sauce until smooth.
   Weeks 5–7: Chop 2 ounces cooked turkey and top with 2 tablespoons sauce.
   Weeks 8+: Serve 2–4 ounces cooked turkey topped with 2 tablespoons sauce.

▶ **FOR OTHERS:**
   Serve 4 ounces cooked turkey topped with 2 tablespoons sauce.

Calories: 172, **Protein:** 25 g, **Fat:** 5 g, **Carbohydrates:** 5 g, **Cholesterol:** 80 mg, **Fiber:** 1 g, **Sodium:** 102 mg

Turkey Curry

I'll admit, I was not a big fan of curries, until a friend who had lived in India made one for me. I tweaked her recipe to make it a bit lighter and quicker.

Canola oil or other neutral-flavor cooking spray

1 medium yellow onion, chopped

3 garlic cloves, minced

1 pound skinless, boneless turkey breast, cut into 1-inch cubes

1 tablespoon grated fresh ginger, or 1½ teaspoons ground

1 teaspoon sweet paprika

1 teaspoon curry powder

½ teaspoon ground cumin

½ teaspoon ground cinnamon

1 (15-ounce) can low-sodium crushed tomatoes

½ cup unsweetened light coconut milk

½ cup plain, fat-free yogurt

½ cup golden raisins, roughly chopped

1. Spray a large skillet with cooking spray. Heat over medium-high heat until it shimmers.
2. Add onion and garlic and cook until soft, about 4 minutes.
3. Stir in turkey breast and cook until golden all over, 3 to 5 minutes.
4. Sprinkle turkey mixture with spices, then add tomatoes and coconut milk, lower heat, and simmer for 5 to 7 minutes.
5. Stir in yogurt and raisins and simmer for 5 more minutes.

Makes 4 servings

SERVING GUIDELINES

▶ **FOR GASTRIC SLEEVE AND BYPASS:**
Week 1: Liquid diet.
Weeks 2–3: Puree 2 ounces cooked turkey curry.
Weeks 4–7: Chop 2 ounces cooked turkey curry.
Weeks 8+: Serve 2–4 ounces cooked turkey curry.

▶ **FOR BPD-DS:**
Week 1: Liquid diet.
Weeks 2–3: Puree 2 ounces cooked turkey curry.
Weeks 4–7: Chop 2 ounces cooked turkey curry.
Weeks 8+: Serve 2–4 ounces cooked turkey curry.

▶ **FOR LAP-BAND:**
Week 1: Liquid diet.
Weeks 2–3: Puree 2 ounces cooked turkey curry.
Weeks 4–7: Chop 2 ounces cooked turkey curry.
Weeks 8+: Serve 2–4 ounces cooked turkey curry.

▶ **FOR OTHERS:**
Serve 4 ounces cooked turkey curry.

Calories: 259, **Protein:** 30 g, **Fat:** 1 g, **Carbohydrates:** 29 g, **Cholesterol:** 69 mg, **Fiber:** 4 g, **Sodium:** 209 mg

Sweet-and-Sour Stuffed Cabbage

Is this your grandma's stuffed cabbage recipe? Kinda-sorta, but not exactly. We omitted the rice and added a citrus tang to the sweet-and-sour sauce.

Filling:

1 pound lean ground turkey
½ cup grated low-fat Swiss cheese
½ cup fat-free ricotta cheese
¼ cup egg substitute
½ cup minced onion
⅛ teaspoon cayenne pepper
⅛ teaspoon freshly ground black pepper

16 large green cabbage leaves, steamed until soft

Sweet-and-Sour Sauce (makes approximately 1 cup):

Canola cooking spray
¼ cup minced onion
1½ teaspoons minced fresh ginger
1½ teaspoons tomato paste
1 (8-ounce) can tomato sauce (no salt added)
2 tablespoons fresh orange juice
1½ teaspoons red wine vinegar
1 packet artificial sweetener (Splenda or Truvia)

1. *To make filling:* In a large bowl, combine all filling ingredients and mix well.
2. *To form cabbage rolls:* Place cabbage leaves on countertop or cutting board. Using a large spoon, place a rounded mound of turkey mixture ¼ inch from edge of each cabbage leaf. Fold top and bottom edges over filling, then starting with filled edge, roll up tightly (you may need to use a toothpick to secure each roll).
3. *To make sauce:* In a large nonstick lidded skillet, heat cooking spray over medium heat until hot but not smoking. Sauté onion until just soft but not brown, add ginger, and stir for 30 seconds. Add all other sauce ingredients and simmer for 5 minutes.
4. *To cook cabbage rolls:* Place rolls in simmering sauce, cover, and cook over medium-low heat for 20 minutes.

Makes 4 servings (16 rolls)

SERVING GUIDELINES

▸ **FOR GASTRIC SLEEVE AND BYPASS:**
Week 1: Liquid diet.
Weeks 2–4: Puree 1 or 2 cooked cabbage rolls
with 2 tablespoons sauce.
Weeks 5+: Serve 2–4 cooked cabbage rolls with 2
tablespoons sauce.

▸ **FOR BPD-DS:**
Week 1: Liquid diet.
Weeks 2–3: Puree 1 or 2 cooked cabbage rolls
with 2 tablespoons sauce.
Weeks 4+: Serve 2–4 cooked cabbage rolls with 2
tablespoons sauce.

▸ **FOR LAP-BAND:**
Week 1: Liquid diet.
Weeks 2–4: Puree 1 or 2 cooked cabbage rolls
with 2 tablespoons sauce.
Weeks 5+: Serve 2–4 cooked cabbage rolls with 2
tablespoons sauce.

▸ **FOR OTHERS:**
Serve 4 cooked cabbage rolls with sauce.

Cabbage:

Calories: 328, **Protein:** 46 g, **Fat:** 6 g, **Carbohydrates:** 26 g, **Cholesterol:** 73 mg, **Fiber:** 6 g, **Sodium:** 264 mg

Sweet-and-Sour Sauce (2 tablespoons):

Calories: 8, **Protein:** 0 g, **Fat:** 0 g, **Carbohydrates:** 2 g, **Cholesterol:** 0 mg, **Fiber:** 0 g, **Sodium:** 7 mg

Asian Turkey-Filled Cabbage Dumplings

Michele and I challenged ourselves to come up with a recipe for dumplings that doesn't contain a lot of carbs, and this delicious concoction made the cut. We experimented until we discovered that cabbage cooked very soft works the same way Asian wrapper dough does.

Dumplings:

3 tablespoons egg white substitute

2 tablespoons light soy sauce

2 tablespoons minced fresh ginger

2 garlic cloves, minced

1 teaspoon sesame oil

1 small jalapeño pepper, seeded and minced

2 packets artificial sweetener (Splenda or Truvia)

1 pound lean ground turkey breast

⅔ cup minced scallion (white and green parts)

1 pound (16 large) green cabbage leaves, steamed until very soft

1 cup water

Dipping Sauce (makes approximately 1 cup):

¾ cup light soy sauce

¼ cup rice vinegar

2 teaspoons red pepper flakes, or to taste

1 teaspoon sesame oil

1. *To make dumplings:* In a large bowl, whisk egg white substitute until frothy, then whisk in soy sauce, ginger, garlic, sesame oil, jalapeño, and sweetener. Add turkey and scallions and mix until well combined.

2. Place 1 cabbage leaf on a flat surface, either a countertop or a cutting board. Spoon 2 tablespoons of turkey mixture in center of leaf, fold sides of leaf over filling, then fold top and bottom of leaf over sides (you may need to use a toothpick to hold dumpling closed). Repeat until you have filled all cabbage leaves.

3. In a large pot or lidded skillet with a steamer insert or a separate steamer basket, bring water to a boil. Place dumplings into steamer, cover, and steam for 15 minutes.

4. *To make sauce:* In a small bowl, combine all sauce ingredients and let stand at room temperature for 10 to 20 minutes.

Makes 4 servings (16 dumplings)

SERVING GUIDELINES

► **FOR GASTRIC SLEEVE AND BYPASS:**
  Week 1: Liquid diet.
  Weeks 2–4: Puree 1–2 steamed dumplings with 2
    tablespoons sauce until smooth.
  Weeks 5+: Serve 2–4 steamed dumplings with 2
    tablespoons dipping sauce.

► **FOR BPD-DS:**
  Week 1: Liquid diet.
  Weeks 2–3: Puree 1–2 steamed dumplings with 2
    tablespoons sauce until smooth.
  Weeks 4+: Serve 2–4 steamed dumplings with 2
    tablespoons dipping sauce.

► **FOR LAP-BAND:**
  Week 1: Liquid diet.
  Weeks 2–4: Puree 1–2 steamed dumplings with 2
    tablespoons sauce until smooth.
  Weeks 5+: Serve 2–4 steamed dumplings with 2
    tablespoons dipping sauce.

► **FOR OTHERS:**
  Serve 4 steamed dumplings with dipping sauce.

Dumplings:

Calories: 191, **Protein:** 32 g, **Fat:** 3 g, **Carbohydrates:** 10 g, **Cholesterol:** 55 mg, **Fiber:** 4 g, **Sodium:** 399 mg

Dipping Sauce (2 tablespoons):

Calories: 15, **Protein:** 1 g, **Fat:** 0 g, **Carbohydrates:** 2 g, **Cholesterol:** 0 mg, **Fiber:** 0 g, **Sodium:** 407 mg

Szechuan Turkey and Eggplant

Authentic? Sure. Spicy? You bet. No one who tastes this dish will ever guess that this is a low-fat, low-calorie version.

3 tablespoons egg white substitute
¼ cup light soy sauce
2 tablespoons minced fresh ginger
2 garlic cloves, minced
1 teaspoon sesame oil
1 tablespoon red pepper flakes
2 packets artificial sweetener
   (Splenda or Truvia)
1 pound lean ground turkey breast
⅔ cup minced scallion
   (white and green parts)
Cooking spray
½ cup chopped onion
2 cups cubed fresh eggplant
1 small jalapeño pepper, seeded and
   minced
1 cup shredded green cabbage
¼ cup water
1 tablespoon rice vinegar

1. In a large bowl, whisk egg white until frothy, then whisk in 2 tablespoons soy sauce, ginger, half of minced garlic, sesame oil, red pepper flakes, and sweetener. Add turkey and scallion and mix until well combined.
2. Coat a large nonstick lidded skillet with cooking spray and heat until hot but not smoking. Sauté onion and remaining minced garlic for about 2 minutes, or until soft.
3. Stir in eggplant, jalapeño, cabbage, water, remaining 2 tablespoons soy sauce, and rice vinegar, bring to a boil, then cover and lower heat. Simmer for 10 minute, or until eggplant is tender.
4. Add turkey mixture, stirring to combine well. Increase heat to medium and cook for 10 minutes, uncovered, or until turkey is cooked through.

Makes 4 servings

SERVING GUIDELINES

▶ **FOR GASTRIC SLEEVE AND BYPASS:**
  Week 1: Liquid diet.
  Weeks 2–4: Puree ¼–½ cup cooked turkey-eggplant until smooth.
  Weeks 5+: Serve ¼–½ cup cooked turkey-eggplant as is.

▶ **FOR BPD-DS:**
  Week 1: Liquid diet.
  Weeks 2–3: Puree ¼–½ cup cooked turkey-eggplant until smooth.
  Weeks 4+: Serve ½–1 cup cooked turkey-eggplant as is.

▶ **FOR LAP-BAND:**
  Week 1: Liquid diet.
  Weeks 2–4: Puree ¼–½ cup cooked turkey-eggplant until smooth.
  Weeks 5+: Serve ¼–½ cup cooked turkey-eggplant as is.

▶ **FOR OTHERS:**
  Serve 1 cup cooked turkey-eggplant as is.

Calories: 196, **Protein:** 31, **Fat:** 3 g, **Carbohydrates:** 11 g, **Cholesterol:** 55 mg, **Fiber:** 3 g, **Sodium:** 644

Teriyaki Turkey Burgers

Satisfy your craving for Japanese flavor with this delicious way to dress up a burger.

1 pound lean ground turkey breast

¼ cup chopped scallion
   (white and green parts)

1 garlic clove, minced

1 teaspoon minced fresh ginger

¼ teaspoon freshly ground black pepper

Canola cooking spray

¼ cup light soy sauce

2 tablespoons rice vinegar

¼ cup dry sherry

1 packet artificial sweetener
   (Splenda or Truvia)

1 cup chopped onion

¼ teaspoon sesame oil

1. In a bowl, combine turkey, scallions, garlic, ginger, and pepper; then, divide mixture into four equal patties.

2. Coat bottom of a medium nonstick skillet with cooking spray and heat over medium heat until hot but not smoking. Cook burgers for 4 minutes on each side, or until cooked through. Remove burgers from pan and keep warm.

3. Pour soy sauce, rice vinegar, and sherry into pan and stir, scraping up any browned bits. Add sweetener and onion and simmer for 5 to 7 minutes, or until onion is soft. Stir in sesame oil.

Makes 4 servings

SERVING GUIDELINES

► **FOR GASTRIC SLEEVE AND BYPASS:**
   Week 1: Liquid diet.
   Weeks 2–3: Puree ½ cooked burger (2 ounces) with 2 tablespoons sauce.
   Weeks 4–7: Chop ½ cooked burger and top with 2 tablespoons sauce.
   Weeks 8+: Serve ½–1 cooked burger topped with 2 tablespoons sauce.

► **FOR BPD-DS:**
   Week 1: Liquid diet.
   Weeks 2–3: Puree ½ cooked burger (2 ounces) with 2 tablespoons sauce.
   Weeks 4+: Serve ½–1 cooked burger topped with 2 tablespoons sauce.

► **FOR LAP-BAND:**
   Week 1: Liquid diet.
   Weeks 2–3: Puree ½ cooked burger (2 ounces) with 2 tablespoons sauce.
   Weeks 4–7: Chop ½ cooked burger and top with 2 tablespoons sauce.
   Weeks 8+: Serve ½–1 cooked burger topped with 2 tablespoons sauce.

► **FOR OTHERS:**
   Serve 4 ounces cooked burger topped with 2 tablespoons sauce.

Calories: 174, **Protein:** 29 g, **Fat:** 2 g, **Carbohydrates:** 7 g, **Cholesterol:** 55 mg, **Fiber:** 1 g, **Sodium:** 620 mg

Korean Barbecue Meatballs and Sauce

Here's a tasty change from meatballs in tomato sauce—it's a little sweet, a little spicy, and altogether delicious.

Meatballs:

1 pound lean ground turkey

¼ cup egg substitute

¼ cup gluten-free unseasoned panko (crispy Japanese-style bread crumbs)

1 garlic clove, minced

Cooking spray

Sauce:

½ cup low-sodium soy sauce

½ cup unsweetened applesauce

2 tablespoons rice vinegar

2 teaspoons minced fresh ginger, or 1 teaspoon ground

3 green onions or scallions, minced

3 garlic cloves, minced

2 teaspoons sesame oil

½ teaspoon crushed red pepper flakes, or more to taste

2 packets Splenda or Truvia

1. *To make meatballs:* In a large bowl, mix all meatball ingredients until well blended. Form into golf ball–size meatballs.

2. Spray a large skillet with cooking spray and heat over medium-high heat until it shimmers.

3. Sauté meatballs until browned on all sides and remove from pan.

4. *To make sauce:* Combine all sauce ingredients in a medium bowl and whisk until sweetener is dissolved.

5. Wipe skillet and pour in sauce mixture. Cook over medium heat until sauce starts to reduce and thicken, 10 to 15 minutes.

6. Add meatballs to sauce, stir, and simmer until well coated and heated through.

Makes 4 servings

SERVING GUIDELINES

- **FOR GASTRIC SLEEVE AND BYPASS:**
  Week 1: Liquid diet.
  Weeks 2–3: Puree 2 ounces cooked meatballs
  with 2 tablespoons sauce.
  Weeks 4–7: Chop 2 ounces cooked meatballs and
  top with 2 tablespoons sauce.
  Weeks 8+: Serve 2–4 ounces cooked meatballs
  with 2 tablespoons sauce.

- **FOR BPD-DS:**
  Week 1: Liquid diet.
  Weeks 2–3: Puree 2 ounces cooked meatballs
  with 2 tablespoons sauce.
  Weeks 4–7: Chop 2 ounces cooked meatballs and
  top with 2 tablespoons sauce.
  Weeks 8+: Serve 2–4 ounces cooked meatballs
  with 2 tablespoons sauce.

- **FOR LAP-BAND:**
  Week 1: Liquid diet.
  Weeks 2–3: Puree 2 ounces cooked meatballs
  with 2 tablespoons sauce.
  Weeks 4–7: Chop 2 ounces cooked meatballs and
  top with 2 tablespoons sauce.
  Weeks 8+: Serve 2–4 ounces cooked meatballs
  with 2 tablespoons sauce.

- **FOR OTHERS:**
  Serve 4 ounces cooked meatballs with sauce.

Calories: 197, **Protein:** 22 g, **Fat:** 5 g, **Carbohydrates:** 19 g, **Cholesterol:** 117 mg, **Fiber:** 1 g, **Sodium:** 1,149 mg

Turkey Loaf with Horseradish Sauce

It's hard to believe that turkey loaf can be so light and moist. We top it with a bold, creamy horseradish sauce. Of course, you could also try it with our Quick Tomato Sauce (page 193), Garlic Sauce (page 186), or Tikka Yogurt Sauce (page 197). Go ahead, experiment.

Turkey Loaf:
1 pound ground turkey
1 (6-ounce) can tomato juice
2 tablespoons dried parsley flakes
1 tablespoon dried celery flakes
1 tablespoon dried onion flakes
¼ cup egg substitute, lightly beaten
1 teaspoon freshly ground black pepper
Cooking spray

Horseradish Sauce
(makes approximately 1 cup):
1 cup fat-free sour cream
3 tablespoons concentrated chicken broth
2 teaspoons sweet paprika
2 tablespoons prepared horseradish

1. Preheat oven to 350°F.
2. *To make turkey loaf:* In a large bowl, combine turkey, tomato juice, parsley, celery flakes, onion flakes, egg substitute, and pepper and mix well.
3. Coat a baking pan with cooking spray. Mound turkey mixture in center of pan to form a loaf and bake for 1 hour.
4. *To make sauce:* Combine all sauce ingredients.

Makes 4 servings

SERVING GUIDELINES

▶ **FOR GASTRIC SLEEVE AND BYPASS:**
   Week 1: Liquid diet.
   Weeks 2–4: Puree 2 ounces cooked turkey loaf with 2 tablespoons sauce until smooth.
   Weeks 5–7: Chop 2 ounces cooked turkey loaf and serve with 2 tablespoons sauce.
   Weeks 8+: Serve 2–4 ounces cooked turkey loaf with 2 tablespoons sauce.

▶ **FOR BPD-DS:**
   Weeks 1: Liquid diet.
   Weeks 2–3: Puree 2 ounces cooked turkey loaf with 2 tablespoons sauce until smooth.
   Weeks 4+: Serve 2–4 ounces cooked turkey loaf with 2 tablespoons sauce.

▶ **FOR LAP-BAND:**
   Week 1: Liquid diet.
   Weeks 2–4: Puree 2 ounces cooked turkey loaf with 2 tablespoons sauce until smooth.
   Weeks 5–7: Chop 2 ounces cooked turkey loaf and serve with 2 tablespoons sauce.
   Weeks 8+: Serve 2–4 ounces cooked turkey loaf with 2 tablespoons sauce.

▶ **FOR OTHERS:**
   Serve 4 ounces cooked turkey loaf with 2 tablespoons sauce.

Turkey Loaf:

Calories: 152, **Protein:** 30 g, **Fat:** 2 g, **Carbohydrates:** 5 g, **Cholesterol:** 55 mg, **Fiber:** 1 g, **Sodium:** 117 mg

Horseradish Sauce (2 tablespoons):

Calories: 24, **Protein:** 1 g, **Fat:** 1 g, **Carbohydrates:** 4 g, **Cholesterol:** 54 mg, **Fiber:** 0 g, **Sodium:** 202 mg

Sausage and Mushrooms with Broccoli Rabe

Talk about peasant cooking—this recipe is a combination of bold, gutsy flavors. It's for the real garlic lover, so be prepared.

Olive oil cooking spray
3 Italian-style hot or sweet lean turkey sausages
½ pound large white mushrooms, sliced
6 large garlic cloves, minced
1 bunch broccoli rabe, tough ends cut off, coarsely chopped (about 4 cups)
½ cup low-sodium chicken broth
½ teaspoon red pepper flakes
Salt and pepper to taste

1. In a medium nonstick lidded skillet, heat cooking spray over medium heat until hot but not smoking. Sauté sausages for 10 minutes, turning frequently to brown. Remove sausages from pan and cut into thick slices.
2. Pour off any accumulated fat from pan, re-spray, and sauté mushrooms and garlic until slightly browned.
3. Add chopped broccoli rabe, chicken broth, and red pepper flakes, cover, and steam for 8 to 10 minutes, or until soft.
4. Toss in sausage slices and heat for 5 minutes. Add salt and pepper to taste.

Makes 4 servings

SERVING GUIDELINES

➤ **FOR GASTRIC SLEEVE AND BYPASS:**
   Week 1: Liquid diet.
   Weeks 2–4: Puree ¼–½ cup cooked sausage-mushrooms with 2 tablespoons broccoli rabe until smooth.
   Weeks 5–7: Chop sausages from ¼–½ cup cooked sausage-mushrooms, top with 2 tablespoons broccoli rabe.
   Weeks 8+: Serve ¼–½ cup cooked sausage-mushrooms-broccoli rabe as is.

➤ **FOR BPD-DS:**
   Week 1: Liquid diet.
   Weeks 2–3: Puree ¼–½ cup cooked sausage-mushrooms with 2 tablespoons broccoli rabe until smooth.
   Weeks 4+: Serve ½–1 cup cooked sausage-mushrooms-broccoli rabe as is.

➤ **FOR LAP-BAND:**
   Week 1: Liquid diet.
   Weeks 2–4: Puree ¼–½ cup cooked sausage-mushrooms with 2 tablespoons broccoli rabe until smooth.
   Weeks 5–7: Chop sausages from ¼–½ cup cooked sausage-mushrooms, top with 2 tablespoons broccoli rabe.
   Weeks 8+: Serve ¼–½ cup cooked sausage-mushrooms as is.

➤ **FOR OTHERS:**
   Serve 1 cup cooked sausage-mushrooms-broccoli rabe as is.

Calories: 160, **Protein:** 16 g, **Fat:** 7 g, **Carbohydrates:** 13 g, **Cholesterol:** 41 mg, **Fiber:** 5 g, **Sodium:** 375 mg

Sausage and Peppers Light

This is the real, old-fashioned classic. I just make my own turkey sausage patties instead of using store-bought pork sausage. Serve it alone or over zasta (zucchini pasta).

Sausage patties:

1 pound ground dark meat turkey

1 teaspoon fennel seeds, crushed

½ teaspoon crushed red pepper flakes

1 teaspoon dried oregano

2 garlic cloves, minced

½ teaspoon dried marjoram

1 teaspoon freshly ground black pepper

Olive oil cooking spray

Peppers and sauce:

1 large onion, peeled and sliced

1 large green bell pepper, cored and sliced

1 large red or yellow bell pepper (or a combination), cored and sliced

2 large garlic cloves, minced

½ (6-ounce) can tomato paste, or 3 tablespoons condensed tomato paste

1 (14.5-ounce) can low-sodium crushed or diced tomatoes

1 tablespoon dried basil

1 teaspoon dried oregano

½ teaspoon red pepper flakes, or more to taste

1. *To make sausage patties:* Mix together all sausage ingredients and form into eight patties.
2. Spray a large lidded skillet or Dutch oven with cooking oil, heat over medium-high heat until it shimmers. Add sausage patties and brown on both sides, 5 to 7 minutes.
3. Remove sausages. Pour out any fat in pan and re-spray.
4. *To make peppers and sauce:* Add onion, peppers, and garlic to pan and cook, stirring until onion begins to brown, about 5 minutes.
5. Add tomato paste and cook, stirring, until paste begins to darken.
6. Add canned tomatoes and seasonings and stir well.
7. Add sausage patties back to pan and turn to coat. Cover pan and cook for 20 minutes.

Makes 4 servings

SERVING GUIDELINES

► **FOR GASTRIC SLEEVE AND BYPASS:**
  Week 1: Liquid diet.
  Weeks 2–3: Puree 1 cooked sausage patty with peppers and sauce.
  Weeks 4–7: Chop 1 cooked sausage patty and peppers and top with sauce.
  Weeks 8+: Serve 1–2 cooked sausage patties with peppers and sauce.

► **FOR BPD-DS:**
  Week 1: Liquid diet.
  Weeks 2–3: Puree 1 cooked sausage patty with peppers and sauce.
  Weeks 4+: Serve 1–2 cooked sausage patties with peppers and sauce.

► **FOR LAP-BAND:**
  Week 1: Liquid diet.
  Weeks 2–3: Puree 1 cooked sausage patty with peppers and sauce.
  Weeks 4–7: Chop 1 cooked sausage patty and peppers and top with sauce.
  Weeks 8+: Serve 1–2 cooked sausage patties with peppers and sauce.

► **FOR OTHERS:**
  Serve 2 cooked sausage patties with peppers and sauce.

Calories: 285, **Protein:** 26 g, **Fat:** 10 g, **Carbohydrates:** 24 g, **Cholesterol:** 75 mg, **Fiber:** 7 g, **Sodium:** 135 mg

Quick No-Bean Turkey Chili

This is just a basic chili recipe except for the unexpected touch of cocoa. If you like your chili hotter, use jalapeño or maybe even Jamaican bird's-eye chiles instead of serrano pepper.

Cooking spray
1 medium onion, chopped
1 medium red bell pepper, seeded and
    diced small
1 medium green bell pepper, seeded and
    diced small
1 teaspoon chili powder
½ fresh serrano pepper, split, seeded, and
    minced (optional)
1 teaspoon ground cumin
1 teaspoon unsweetened cocoa powder
½ teaspoon salt
1 teaspoon ground cinnamon
½ teaspoon freshly ground black pepper
1 pound lean ground turkey
1 (28-ounce) can low-sodium whole
    tomatoes, chopped, with juice
1 tablespoon cider vinegar
2 packets artificial sweetener
    (Splenda or Truvia)
½ cup shredded low-fat Cheddar cheese

1. Coat a deep nonstick skillet with cooking spray and heat over medium-high heat. Sauté onion, stirring, until lightly browned, about 5 minutes.
2. Add bell peppers and sauté for about 6 minutes, stirring occasionally, until softened.
3. Add chili powder, minced serrano pepper, cumin, cocoa powder, salt, cinnamon, and black pepper and cook, stirring, for 1 minute.
4. Add turkey and cook, stirring to break up any lumps, for 5 to 7 minutes, or until completely browned.
5. Add tomatoes with juice, cider vinegar, and sweetener and simmer briskly, uncovered, stirring occasionally, until thickened, 15 to 20 minutes.
6. Top each serving with 2 tablespoons Cheddar cheese.

Makes 4 servings

SERVING GUIDELINES

▶ **FOR GASTRIC SLEEVE AND BYPASS:**
   Week 1: Liquid diet.
   Weeks 2–3: Puree 2 ounces cooked chili.
   Weeks 4+: Serve 2–4 ounces cooked chili.

▶ **FOR BPD-DS:**
   Week 1: Liquid diet.
   Weeks 2–3: Puree 2 ounces cooked chili.
   Weeks 4+: Serve 2–4 ounces cooked chili.

▶ **FOR LAP-BAND:**
   Week 1: Liquid diet.
   Weeks 2–3: Puree 2 ounces cooked chili.
   Weeks 4+: Serve 2–4 ounces cooked chili.

▶ **FOR OTHERS:**
   Serve 4 ounces cooked chili.

Calories: 266, **Protein:** 32 g, **Fat:** 5 g, **Carbohydrates:** 14 g, **Cholesterol:** 68 mg, **Fiber:** 4 g, **Sodium:** 478 mg

No-Noodle Zucchini Lasagna

Yes, you can take out the pasta and still make great lasagna. This version is what's known as "white lasagna," which simply means no tomatoes.

½ pound (1 large) zucchini, sliced
vertically into six to eight ⅛-inch-
thick slices
½ teaspoon salt
Olive oil cooking spray
¾ cup chopped onion
2 garlic cloves, minced
2 cups thinly sliced fresh mushrooms
½ pound lean ground turkey breast
½ cup skim milk
1 (10-ounce) package frozen chopped
spinach, thawed, drained, and
squeezed dry
½ cup fat-free ricotta cheese
⅓ cup chopped fresh parsley
⅛ teaspoon ground nutmeg
¼ teaspoon dried oregano
3 tablespoons grated Parmesan cheese
½ cup grated part-skim mozzarella cheese

1. Preheat oven to 400°F.
2. Lay zucchini slices on a double thickness of paper towels, sprinkle with salt, cover with more paper towels, and let stand for 15 minutes.
3. Line a cookie sheet with aluminum foil and spray with cooking spray. Arrange zucchini slices on foil in one layer and bake for 15 minutes. Remove from oven and let cool.
4. Coat bottom of medium skillet with cooking spray and heat over medium heat until hot but not smoking. Brown onion and garlic for 2 minutes; add mushrooms and brown for 2 minutes.
5. Add ground turkey and brown, stirring to break up, for 3 minutes, or until cooked completely. Remove from heat.
6. In a medium saucepan, bring milk to a boil. Remove from heat and stir in spinach, ricotta cheese, parsley, nutmeg, oregano, and 2 tablespoons of Parmesan cheese.
7. Spoon half of spinach mixture into bottom of an 8-inch square baking pan or casserole dish, then layer on half of mushroom-turkey mixture and lay three to four zucchini slices on top. Repeat layers, ending with a zucchini layer. Sprinkle with mozzarella and remaining tablespoon of Parmesan cheese and bake for 40 minutes.

Makes 4 servings

► **Cooking Tip:** If you have any leftovers, this freezes well.

COOKED

► **FOR GASTRIC SLEEVE AND BYPASS:**
  Week 1: Liquid diet.
  Weeks 2–4: Puree ¼–½ cup lasagna until smooth.
  Weeks 5+: Serve ¼–½ cup lasagna as is.

► **FOR BPD-DS:**
  Week 1: Liquid diet.
  Weeks 2–3: Puree ¼–½ cup lasagna until smooth.
  Weeks 4+: Serve ¾–1 cup lasagna as is.

► **FOR LAP-BAND:**
  Week 1: Liquid diet.
  Weeks 2–4: Puree ¼–½ cup lasagna until smooth.
  Weeks 5+: Serve ¼–½ cup lasagna as is.

► **FOR OTHERS:**
  Serve 1 cup lasagna as is.

Calories: 238, **Protein:** 30 g, **Fat:** 8 g, **Carbohydrates:** 14 g, **Cholesterol:** 49 mg, **Fiber:** 4 g, **Sodium:** 1,341 mg

Un-Pasta Lasagna with Tomato Sauce

This is another one of those clever zucchini lasagnas, but this one is bursting with tomatoes and turkey sausage, and lots of real southern Italian flavor.

½ pound large zucchini, sliced vertically ¼ inch thick (6 to 8 slices)
½ teaspoon salt
Olive oil cooking spray
½ pound sweet or hot Italian-style low-fat turkey sausages (about 2), removed from casings
1 cup chopped onion
2 garlic cloves, minced
2 tablespoons tomato paste
1 (14.5-ounce) can diced tomatoes, drained
½ cup dry red wine
½ packet artificial sweetener (Splenda or Truvia)
1 tablespoon chopped fresh basil, or 1½ teaspoons dried
½ cup shredded part-skim mozzarella cheese
½ cup fat-free ricotta cheese
3 tablespoons grated Parmesan cheese
Salt and pepper to taste

1. Preheat oven to 400°F.
2. Lay zucchini slices on a double thickness of paper towels, sprinkle with salt, cover with more paper towels, and let stand for 15 minutes.
3. Line a cookie sheet with aluminum foil and spray with cooking spray. Lay zucchini slices on foil in one layer and bake for 15 minutes, then remove from oven and let cool.
4. Coat bottom of a large nonstick skillet with cooking spray. Sauté sausage meat for 5 minutes over medium heat. Remove from skillet and discard any fat in pan.
5. Re-spray pan and, over medium-high heat, brown onion and garlic for 3 minutes.
6. Add tomato paste to onion and cook, stirring, until tomato paste begins to darken, about 1 minute.
7. Add diced tomatoes, wine, sweetener, and basil and bring to a boil; then, lower heat and simmer for 5 minutes.
8. In a small bowl, combine mozzarella and ricotta cheeses with 2 tablespoons of Parmesan; stir in cooked sausage.
9. Spoon one third of tomato sauce in bottom of an 8-inch square baking pan or casserole dish. Lay three to four slices of zucchini on top, then layer on half of cheese-sausage mixture. Repeat layers, ending with sauce layer. Sprinkle with remaining tablespoon Parmesan cheese and bake for 40 minutes.
10. Serve and add salt and pepper to taste.

Makes 4 servings

➤ **Cooking Tip:** If you have any leftovers, this freezes well.

SERVING GUIDELINES

➤ **FOR GASTRIC SLEEVE AND BYPASS:**
  Week 1: Liquid diet.
  Weeks 2–4: Puree ¼–½ cup lasagna until smooth.
  Weeks 5+: Serve ¼–½ cup lasagna as is.

➤ **FOR BPD-DS:**
  Week 1: Liquid diet.
  Weeks 2–3: Puree ¼–½ cup lasagna until smooth.
  Weeks 4+: Serve ¾–1 cup lasagna as is.

➤ **FOR LAP-BAND:**
  Week 1: Liquid diet.
  Weeks 2–4: Puree ¼–½ cup lasagna until smooth.
  Weeks 5+: Serve ¼–½ cup lasagna as is.

➤ **FOR OTHERS:**
  Serve 1 cup lasagna as is.

Calories: 301, **Protein:** 25 g, **Fat:** 13 g, **Carbohydrates:** 19 g, **Cholesterol:** 65 mg, **Fiber:** 3 g, **Sodium:** 1,740 mg

Sausage and Ricotta Giardiniera

This is a rustic Italian one-dish meal that involves a lot of chopping and substantial cooking time, but it's even better when cooked a day ahead and reheated.

Olive oil cooking spray
½ pound Italian-style hot or sweet lean turkey sausages, removed from casings
½ cup coarsely chopped onion
2 large garlic cloves, minced
½ pound fresh white mushrooms, cut into eighths
1 small zucchini, cut into coarse cubes (about 1 cup)
1 small bell pepper, seeded and cut up coarsely (about 1 cup)
1 (14.5-ounce) can low-sodium diced tomatoes
½ cup dry red wine
1 tablespoon minced fresh basil, or 1½ teaspoons dried
1 teaspoon red pepper flakes
½ cup fat-free ricotta cheese
¼ cup minced or shredded part-skim mozzarella cheese
Salt and pepper to taste

1. In a 4- to 5-quart pot, heat cooking spray over medium-high heat until hot but not smoking. Sauté sausage meat for 5 minutes, or until cooked through, stirring to break up lumps. Remove from pot with slotted spoon and pour off fat.
2. Add onion, garlic, and mushrooms and cook for about 3 minutes, or until onion and garlic are just translucent.
3. Stir in sausage, zucchini, bell pepper, tomatoes, wine, basil, and red pepper flakes, then cover pot and cook over low heat for 1½ hours.
4. Stir in ricotta and mozzarella cheeses and salt and pepper to taste; cover and simmer for 5 minutes.

Makes 8 servings

SERVING GUIDELINES

- ▸ **FOR GASTRIC SLEEVE AND BYPASS:**
  Week 1: Liquid diet.
  Weeks 2–4: Puree ½ cup cooked sausage-cheese until smooth.
  Weeks 5+: Serve ½ cup cooked sausage-cheese as is.

- ▸ **FOR BPD-DS:**
  Week 1: Liquid diet.
  Weeks 2–3: Puree ½ cup cooked sausage-cheese until smooth.
  Weeks 4+: Serve ½–1 cup cooked sausage-cheese as is.

- ▸ **FOR LAP-BAND:**
  Week 1: Liquid diet.
  Weeks 2–4: Puree ½ cup cooked sausage-cheese until smooth.
  Weeks 5+: Serve ½ cup cooked sausage-cheese as is.

- ▸ **FOR OTHERS:**
  Serve 1 cup cooked sausage-cheese.

Calories: 252, **Protein:** 21 g, **Fat:** 9 g, **Carbohydrates:** 19 g, **Cholesterol:** 55 mg, **Fiber:** 4 g, **Sodium:** 670 mg

Braised Pork Tenderloin

This is a savory way to cook a very mild, lean cut of meat. Instead of slicing the tenderloin before cooking, you marinate it to flavor and tenderize it, then quickly braise it.

1½ cups chopped leeks, rinsed well
1 cup dry white wine
1 tablespoon Dijon mustard
Brown-sugar artificial sweetener
   (1 teaspoon equivalent)
2 garlic cloves, minced
¼ tablespoon ground thyme
1 tablespoon prepared horseradish
Salt and pepper to taste
1 pound lean pork tenderloin
Canola cooking spray

1. In a large bowl, combine leeks, ½ cup of wine, mustard, sweetener, garlic, thyme, horseradish, salt, and pepper and pour into a large resealable plastic bag.
2. Add pork tenderloin to bag, seal it, and shake to coat completely. Chill in refrigerator for 2½ hours.
3. Remove pork from bag, reserving marinade. Coat bottom of large nonstick lidded skillet with cooking spray and heat over medium-high heat until hot but not smoking. Sear pork for 2 minutes on each side.
4. Pour remaining ½ cup of wine into reserved marinade in bag, shake well, and pour over pork.
5. Lower heat to medium-low, cover skillet, and braise for 15 to 20 minutes, or until pork is cooked through. Remove pork, slice thinly, and keep warm.
6. Simmer sauce for 3 minutes to reduce slightly.

Makes 4 servings

SERVING GUIDELINES

► **FOR GASTRIC SLEEVE AND BYPASS:**
   Week 1: Liquid diet.
   Weeks 2–4: Puree 2 ounces cooked pork with 2 tablespoons sauce.
   Weeks 5–7: Chop 2 ounces cooked pork and top with sauce.
   Weeks 8+: Serve 2–4 ounces cooked pork topped with sauce.

► **FOR BPD-DS:**
   Week 1: Liquid diet.
   Weeks 2–3: Puree 2 ounces cooked pork with 2 tablespoons sauce.
   Weeks 4+: Serve 3–4 ounces cooked pork topped with sauce.

► **FOR LAP-BAND:**
   Week 1: Liquid diet.
   Weeks 2–4: Puree 2 ounces cooked pork with 2 tablespoons sauce.
   Weeks 5–7: Chop 2 ounces cooked pork and top with sauce.
   Weeks 8+: Serve 2–4 ounces cooked pork topped with sauce.

► **FOR OTHERS:**
   Serve 4 ounces cooked pork topped with sauce.

Calories: 234, **Protein:** 24 g, **Fat:** 8 g, **Carbohydrates:** 7 g, **Cholesterol:** 0 mg, **Fiber:** 1 g, **Sodium:** 126 mg

Braised Pork with Apples and Onions

This recipe is the epitome of autumn to me. It takes the juicy spiciness of baked apples and combines them with the tenderest pork.

1 pound pork tenderloin

Olive oil cooking spray

2 garlic cloves, minced

¼ teaspoon ground nutmeg

1 tablespoon ground fresh grated ginger, or 2 teaspoons ground

1 large onion, cut into ½-inch wedges (about 1½ cups)

2 medium Granny Smith apples, peeled, cored, and cut into ½-inch wedges

2 packets artificial sweetener (Splenda or Truvia)

½ teaspoon ground cinnamon

½ cup water

1. Preheat oven to 350°F.
2. Place pork tenderloin in a baking pan that has been coated with cooking spray.
3. In a small bowl, combine garlic, nutmeg, and ginger and rub onto pork.
4. Surround tenderloin with alternating wedges of onion and apple. Spray onion and apple wedges with cooking spray, sprinkle with sweetener and cinnamon, and pour water over onions and apples.
5. Cover with foil and bake for 20 minutes. Remove foil and bake for 10 minutes more.
6. Slice meat thinly and serve.

Makes 4 servings

SERVING GUIDELINES

▶ **FOR GASTRIC SLEEVE AND BYPASS:**
   Week 1: Liquid diet.
   Weeks 2–4: Puree 2 ounces cooked pork with ¼ cup cooked apples and onions.
   Weeks 5–7: Chop 2 ounces pork and top with ¼ cup apples and onions.
   Weeks 8+: Serve 2–4 ounces pork topped with ¼ cup apples and onions.

▶ **FOR BPD-DS:**
   Week 1: Liquid diet.
   Weeks 2–3: Puree 2 ounces cooked pork with ¼ cup cooked apples and onions.
   Weeks 4+: Serve 3–4 ounces pork topped with ¼ cup apples and onions.

▶ **FOR LAP-BAND:**
   Week 1: Liquid diet.
   Weeks 2–4: Puree 2 ounces cooked pork with ¼ cup cooked apples and onions.
   Weeks 5–7: Chop 2 ounces pork and top with ¼ cup apples and onions.
   Weeks 8+: Serve 2–4 ounces pork topped with ¼ cup apples and onions.

▶ **FOR OTHERS:**
   Serve 4 ounces pork topped with ¼ cup cooked apples and onions.

Calories: 233, **Protein:** 24 g, **Fat:** 7 g, **Carbohydrates:** 17 g, **Cholesterol:** 0 mg, **Fiber:** 3 g, **Sodium:** 56 mg

Indonesian Braised Pork

Sort of a cross between Asian and Indian, this recipe is surprisingly light and luscious.

1 pound lean pork tenderloin
Canola cooking spray
½ cup chopped shallots
½ teaspoon Asian chili paste with garlic
1 tablespoon minced fresh ginger
1½ tablespoons light soy sauce
1 cup light unsweetened coconut milk
2 tablespoons fresh lime juice

1. Slice tenderloin in ½-inch-thick slices.
2. In a medium nonstick lidded skillet, heat cooking spray over medium-high heat. Brown pork for about 1 minute on each side. Add shallots and sauté until golden.
3. In a small bowl, mix chili paste, ginger, soy sauce, and coconut milk. Add to pan, cover, then lower heat and simmer, turning meat occasionally, for about 2 minutes, or until it is cooked through.
4. Add lime juice, stir, and simmer for 1 more minute.

Makes 4 servings

SERVING GUIDELINES

▶ **FOR GASTRIC SLEEVE AND BYPASS:**
  Week 1: Liquid diet.
  Weeks 2–4: Puree 2 ounces cooked pork with 2 tablespoons sauce.
  Weeks 5–7: Chop 2 ounces cooked pork and top with sauce.
  Weeks 8+: Serve 2–4 ounces cooked pork topped with sauce.

▶ **FOR BPD-DS:**
  Week 1: Liquid diet.
  Weeks 2–3: Puree 2 ounces cooked pork with 2 tablespoons sauce.
  Weeks 4+: Serve 3–4 ounces cooked pork topped with sauce.

▶ **FOR LAP-BAND:**
  Week 1: Liquid diet.
  Weeks 2–4: Puree 2 ounces cooked pork with 2 tablespoons sauce.
  Weeks 5–7: Chop 2 ounces cooked pork and top with sauce.
  Weeks 8+: Serve 2–4 ounces cooked pork topped with sauce.

▶ **FOR OTHERS:**
  Serve 4 ounces cooked pork topped with sauce.

Calories: 334, **Protein:** 24 g, **Fat:** 11 g, **Carbohydrates:** 7 g, **Cholesterol:** 0 mg, **Fiber:** 0 g, **Sodium:** 295 mg

Madeira-Glazed Pork

Pork medallions glazed with a subtly sweet yet piquant sauce really make an elegant entrée. The unexpected ingredient? Vanilla.

1 pound pork tenderloin
Butter-flavored cooking spray
¾ cup thinly sliced shallots
¾ cup Madeira wine
¼ teaspoon vanilla extract
2 tablespoons balsamic vinegar
Brown-sugar artificial sweetener
  (1 teaspoon equivalent)
Salt and pepper to taste

1. Slice tenderloin into ½-inch slices.
2. In a large nonstick skillet, heat cooking spray and sauté pork over medium heat for 4 minutes, turning once. Remove from pan and keep warm.
3. Add shallots to pan and sauté for 3 minutes.
4. Add wine and vanilla to pan, stirring to scrape up any browned bits. Lower heat and simmer for 10 minutes, or until liquid is reduced slightly.
5. Stir in balsamic vinegar and sweetener, return pork and any accumulated juices to pan, and turn once to coat. Add salt and pepper to taste.

Makes 4 servings

SERVING GUIDELINES

► **FOR GASTRIC SLEEVE AND BYPASS:**
   Week 1: Liquid diet.
   Weeks 2–4: Puree 2 ounces cooked pork with 2 tablespoons sauce.
   Weeks 5–7: Chop 2 ounces cooked pork and top with sauce.
   Weeks 8+: Serve 2–4 ounces cooked pork topped with sauce.

► **FOR BPD-DS:**
   Week 1: Liquid diet.
   Weeks 2–3: Puree 2 ounces cooked pork with 2 tablespoons sauce.
   Weeks 4+: Serve 3–4 ounces cooked pork topped with sauce.

► **FOR LAP-BAND:**
   Week 1: Liquid diet.
   Weeks 2–4: Puree 2 ounces cooked pork with 2 tablespoons sauce.
   Weeks 5–7: Chop 2 ounces cooked pork and top with sauce.
   Weeks 8+: Serve 2–4 ounces cooked pork topped with sauce.

► **FOR OTHERS:**
   Serve 4 ounces cooked pork topped with sauce.

Calories: 259, **Protein:** 24 g, **Fat:** 7 g, **Carbohydrates:** 12 g, **Cholesterol:** 0 mg, **Fiber:** 0 g, **Sodium:** 176 mg

Medallions of Pork with Mushrooms

A creamy sauce with the tang of mustard turns ordinary pork into a dish that tastes special, yet is easy enough for even a workday dinner.

1 pound pork tenderloin
Butter-flavored cooking spray
½ cup thinly sliced shallots
1 cup thinly sliced fresh mushrooms
½ cup dry white wine
2 tablespoons concentrated chicken broth
¼ teaspoon dried thyme
2 teaspoons whole-grain mustard
¼ cup fat-free sour cream
Salt and pepper to taste

1. Slice tenderloin into ½-inch slices.
2. In a medium nonstick skillet, heat cooking spray over medium-high heat until hot but not smoking. Brown pork on both sides, then lower heat and sauté for 3 minutes, until cooked through. Remove pork from pan.
3. Re-spray pan and sauté shallots and mushrooms, stirring until lightly browned.
4. Stir in wine, scraping up any browned bits. Add concentrated chicken broth and thyme and simmer for 2 minutes.
5. Stir in mustard and sour cream and simmer for 1 to 2 minutes. Add pork and any accumulated meat juices and turn pork to coat. Add salt and pepper to taste.

Makes 4 servings

SERVING GUIDELINES

► **FOR GASTRIC SLEEVE AND BYPASS:**
Week 1: Liquid diet.
Weeks 2–4: Puree 2 ounces cooked pork with 2 tablespoons sauce.
Weeks 5–7: Chop 2 ounces cooked pork and top with sauce.
Weeks 8+: Serve 2–4 ounces cooked pork topped with sauce.

► **FOR BPD-DS:**
Week 1: Liquid diet.
Weeks 2–3: Puree 2 ounces cooked pork with 2 tablespoons sauce.
Weeks 4+: Serve 3–4 ounces cooked pork topped with sauce.

► **FOR LAP-BAND:**
Week 1: Liquid diet.
Weeks 2–4: Puree 2 ounces cooked pork with 2 tablespoons sauce.
Weeks 5–7: Chop 2 ounces cooked pork and top with sauce.
Weeks 8+: Serve 2–4 ounces cooked pork topped with sauce.

► **FOR OTHERS:**
Serve 4 ounces cooked pork topped with sauce.

Calories: 232, **Protein:** 25 g, **Fat:** 8 g, **Carbohydrates:** 8 g, **Cholesterol:** 3 mg, **Fiber:** 0 g, **Sodium:** 521 mg

Pork Tenderloin with Fresh Plum Sauce

When we were trying to come up with an Asian-style pork recipe, almost every one we researched contained hoisin sauce (very heavy on sugar). So, we concocted this plum sauce, which not only tastes incredible, but is incredibly versatile as well.

Pork tenderloin:

1 teaspoon paprika
½ teaspoon ground allspice
¼ teaspoon ground nutmeg
½ teaspoon cayenne pepper
1 teaspoon ground ginger
½ teaspoon ground thyme
1 packet artificial sweetener
   (Splenda or Truvia)
1 pound lean pork tenderloin

Fresh Plum Sauce
(makes approximately 1 cup):

Canola cooking spray
½ cup chopped onion
3 large red or purple plums,
   pitted and chopped
1 garlic clove, minced
1 tablespoon tomato paste
½ small jalapeño pepper, seeded and
   minced
1 tablespoon balsamic vinegar
1 tablespoon light soy sauce
Brown-sugar artificial sweetener
   (1 teaspoon equivalent)

1. Preheat oven to 375°F.
2. *To make pork:* In a small bowl, mix all spices and sweetener together to form a dry rub.
3. Rub spice mixture all over tenderloin and bake, uncovered, for 15 minutes.
4. *While pork bakes, make plum sauce:* Coat a nonstick saucepan with cooking spray. Heat over medium heat and sauté onion until just translucent. Add all other sauce ingredients and cook over low heat for 10 minutes until thick. Let cool slightly, pour into food processor, and blend until smooth.
5. Spoon ½ cup of plum sauce onto tenderloin and bake for another 10 minutes.
6. Slice tenderloin thinly on diagonal and serve with remaining sauce.

Makes 4 servings

SERVING GUIDELINES

▸ **FOR GASTRIC SLEEVE AND BYPASS:**
  Week 1: Liquid diet.
  Weeks 2–4: Puree 2 ounces cooked pork with 2 tablespoons sauce.
  Weeks 5–7: Chop 2 ounces cooked pork and top with sauce.
  Weeks 8+: Serve 2–4 ounces cooked pork topped with sauce.

▸ **FOR BPD-DS:**
  Week 1: Liquid diet.
  Weeks 2–3: Puree 2 ounces cooked pork with 2 tablespoons sauce.
  Weeks 4+: Serve 3–4 ounces cooked pork topped with sauce.

▸ **FOR LAP-BAND:**
  Week 1: Liquid diet.
  Weeks 2–4: Puree 2 ounces cooked pork with 2 tablespoons sauce.
  Weeks 5–7: Chop 2 ounces cooked pork and top with sauce.
  Weeks 8+: Serve 2–4 ounces cooked pork topped with sauce.

▸ **FOR OTHERS:**
  Serve 4 ounces cooked pork topped with sauce.

Pork Tenderloin:

Calories: 168, **Protein:** 23 g, **Fat:** 7 g, **Carbohydrates:** 1 g, **Cholesterol:** 0 mg, **Fiber:** 0 g, **Sodium:** 54 mg

Plum Sauce (2 tablespoons):

Calories: 12, **Protein:** 0 g, **Fat:** 0 g, **Carbohydrates:** 3 g, **Cholesterol:** 0 mg, **Fiber:** 32 g, **Sodium:** 49 mg

Pork with Onions and Capers

Capers, those tender little buds that pack a lot of flavor, add an unexpected hint of sharpness to a lovely creamy onion sauce. Drain and rinse jarred capers before using them in this recipe.

1 pound pork tenderloin
Butter-flavored cooking spray
1½ cups thinly sliced onion
½ cup dry vermouth
¼ cup water
2 teaspoons concentrated chicken broth
2 tablespoons capers
¼ cup fat-free sour cream
Salt and pepper to taste

1. Slice tenderloin into ½-inch slices.
2. In a large nonstick skillet, heat cooking spray over medium-high heat until hot but not smoking. Sauté pork for about 2 minutes on each side, then remove from pan.
3. Re-spray pan and add onion. Cook, stirring, for 3 to 4 minutes, or until onion just starts to brown.
4. Add vermouth and water and simmer for 3 to 4 minutes, or until liquid is reduced to about ¼ cup.
5. Stir in concentrated chicken broth and capers. Increase heat to high and bring onion mixture to a boil, then cook until reduced by half.
6. Turn off heat, stir in sour cream, and add sliced pork and any accumulated meat juices back to skillet. Turn pork slices to coat, and serve. Salt and pepper to taste.

Makes 4 servings

SERVING GUIDELINES

► **FOR GASTRIC SLEEVE AND BYPASS:**
  Week 1: Liquid diet.
  Weeks 2–4: Puree 2 ounces cooked pork with 2 tablespoons sauce.
  Weeks 5–7: Chop 2 ounces cooked pork and top with sauce.
  Weeks 8+: Serve 2–4 ounces cooked pork topped with sauce.

► **FOR BPD-DS:**
  Week 1: Liquid diet.
  Weeks 2–3: Puree 2 ounces cooked pork with 2 tablespoons sauce.
  Weeks 4+: Serve 3–4 ounces cooked pork topped with sauce.

► **FOR LAP-BAND:**
  Week 1: Liquid diet.
  Weeks 2–4: Puree 2 ounces cooked pork with 2 tablespoons sauce.
  Weeks 5–7: Chop 2 ounces cooked pork and top with sauce.
  Weeks 8+: Serve 2–4 ounces cooked pork topped with sauce.

► **FOR OTHERS:**
  Serve 4 ounces cooked pork topped with sauce.

Calories: 226, **Protein:** 24 g, **Fat:** 7 g, **Carbohydrates:** 7 g, **Cholesterol:** 3 mg, **Fiber:** 1 g, **Sodium:** 375 mg

Thai Caramel Pork

Like the best Thai recipes, this one has all the tastes—salty, sweet, sour, and hot. It might sound contradictory, but trust me; the way these tastes are combined in this sauce, they complement one another perfectly.

1 cup unsweetened light coconut milk
Brown-sugar artificial sweetener
  (1 teaspoon equivalent)
¼ cup Asian fish sauce
½ cup thinly sliced shallots
½ teaspoon cayenne pepper
Canola cooking spray
1 pound pork tenderloin
1 tablespoon rice vinegar

1. Pour coconut milk and sweetener into a heavy saucepan and simmer, uncovered, over medium-high heat until slightly thickened and light brown.
2. Add fish sauce and shallots, lower heat, and cook, stirring occasionally, for about 5 minutes. Add cayenne and set aside to cool.
3. In a large lidded nonstick skillet, heat cooking spray over medium-high heat until hot but not smoking. Sear pork on one side for about 2 minutes, then turn and sear on other side for 1 minute.
4. Lower heat to medium, cover skillet, and cook pork for 10 to 12 minutes, or until cooked through. Remove pork from pan and slice thinly on the diagonal.
5. Deglaze pan with vinegar, scraping up any browned bits. Add cooled sauce and stir over low heat for 2 minutes. Add pork to coat and turn off heat.

Makes 4 servings

SERVING GUIDELINES

► **FOR GASTRIC SLEEVE AND BYPASS:**
  Week 1: Liquid diet.
  Weeks 2–4: Puree 2 ounces cooked pork with 2 tablespoons sauce.
  Weeks 5–7: Chop 2 ounces cooked pork and top with sauce.
  Weeks 8+: Serve 2–4 ounces cooked pork topped with sauce.

► **FOR BPD-DS:**
  Week 1: Liquid diet.
  Weeks 2–3: Puree 2 ounces cooked pork with 2 tablespoons sauce.
  Weeks 4+: Serve 3–4 ounces cooked pork topped with sauce.

► **FOR LAP-BAND:**
  Week 1: Liquid diet.
  Weeks 2–4: Puree 2 ounces cooked pork with 2 tablespoons sauce.
  Weeks 5–7: Chop 2 ounces cooked pork and top with sauce.
  Weeks 8+: Serve 2–4 ounces cooked pork topped with sauce.

► **FOR OTHERS:**
  Serve 4 ounces cooked pork topped with sauce.

Calories: 229, **Protein:** 24 g, **Fat:** 11 g, **Carbohydrates:** 6 g, **Cholesterol:** 0 mg, **Fiber:** 0 g, **Sodium:** 1,165 mg

Smothered Pork Chops

Here is a way to take a classic southern recipe and make it lower in everything—fat, carbs—except flavor.

4 pork chops, about ½ inch thick, trimmed of fat
1½ cups fat-free buttermilk
2 tablespoons sweet or smoked paprika
½ teaspoon freshly ground black pepper
2 tablespoons onion powder
1 tablespoon garlic powder
1 teaspoon cayenne pepper
Canola cooking spray
2 large onions, sliced
1 garlic clove, minced
1½ cups low-sodium chicken broth
½ cup reduced-fat sour cream
1 teaspoon hot sauce (or to taste)

1. Place pork chops in a large resealable plastic bag.
2. In a bowl, mix together buttermilk with paprika, pepper, onion powder, garlic powder, and cayenne. Pour over pork chops, seal bag, and marinate in refrigerator for 30 minutes.
3. Remove pork chops from bag and pat dry.
4. Spray large skillet with cooking spray and heat over medium-high heat until hot but not smoking. Sauté pork for 2 minutes on one side, turn, and cook for 2 minutes on the other. Remove chops from pan and keep warm.
5. Re-spray pan and heat until shimmering. Add onions and garlic and cook, stirring, for 3 to 5 minutes, or until soft but not browned.
6. Lower heat, pour chicken broth into pan, and simmer for 10 to 12 minutes. Add sour cream and hot sauce and stir until smooth. Add pork chops back to skillet and simmer for 5 minutes.

Makes 4 servings

SERVING GUIDELINES

➤ **FOR GASTRIC SLEEVE AND BYPASS:**
  Week 1: Liquid diet.
  Weeks 2–7: Puree 2 ounces cooked pork with 2 tablespoons sauce.
  Weeks 8+: Serve 2–4 ounces cooked pork with 2 tablespoons sauce.

➤ **FOR BPD-DS:**
  Week 1: Liquid diet.
  Weeks 2–7: Puree 2 ounces cooked pork with 2 tablespoons sauce.
  Weeks 8+: Serve 2–4 ounces cooked pork with 2 tablespoons sauce.

➤ **FOR LAP-BAND:**
  Week 1: Liquid diet.
  Weeks 2–7: Puree 2 ounces cooked pork with 2 tablespoons sauce.
  Weeks 8+: Serve 2–4 ounces cooked pork with 2 tablespoons sauce.

➤ **FOR OTHERS:**
  Serve 4 ounces cooked pork with sauce.

Calories: 293, **Protein:** 30 g, **Fat:** 9 g, **Carbohydrates:** 18 g, **Cholesterol:** 65 mg, **Fiber:** 2 g, **Sodium:** 366 mg

Cider-Glazed Pork Chops

Here is another one of those perfect pairings—pork and apple cider. This simple recipe emphasizes the tang of the fruit, without being too sweet.

Butter-flavored cooking spray
1 pound lean boneless pork chops
1 cup apple cider
Brown-sugar artificial sweetener
   (1 teaspoon equivalent)
1 teaspoon Dijon mustard
½ cup fat-free, low-sodium chicken broth
2 tablespoons cider vinegar

1. In a medium nonstick skillet, heat cooking spray over medium-high heat until hot but not smoking. Sauté pork for 2 minutes on one side, turn, and cook for 2 minutes on the other, then remove chops and keep warm.
2. Stir together cider and sweetener and add to skillet. Simmer, uncovered, for 1 minute; then add mustard, broth, and vinegar, stirring to scrape up any browned bits. Simmer for 5 minutes, or until sauce is slightly thickened.
3. Return chops to pan with any meat juices that have accumulated and turn chops in sauce to coat. Simmer for 2 more minutes over low heat, then serve.

Makes 4 servings

SERVING GUIDELINES

▶ **FOR GASTRIC SLEEVE AND BYPASS:**
Week 1: Liquid diet.
Weeks 2–4: Puree 2 ounces cooked pork with 2 tablespoons sauce.
Weeks 5–7: Chop 2 ounces cooked pork and top with sauce.
Weeks 8+: Serve 2–4 ounces cooked pork topped with sauce.

▶ **FOR BPD-DS:**
Week 1: Liquid diet.
Weeks 2–3: Puree 2 ounces cooked pork with 2 tablespoons sauce.
Weeks 4+: Serve 3–4 ounces cooked pork topped with sauce.

▶ **FOR LAP-BAND:**
Week 1: Liquid diet.
Weeks 2–4: Puree 2 ounces cooked pork with 2 tablespoons sauce.
Weeks 5–7: Chop 2 ounces cooked pork and top with sauce.
Weeks 8+: Serve 2–4 ounces cooked pork topped with sauce.

▶ **FOR OTHERS:**
Serve 4 ounces cooked pork topped with sauce.

Calories: 257, **Protein:** 26 g, **Fat:** 14 g, **Carbohydrates:** 8 g, **Cholesterol:** 0 mg, **Fiber:** 0 g, **Sodium:** 82 mg

Smoked Pork Chops with Pineapple

This is a slightly more sophisticated version of the classic ham steak with pineapple slices—and, yes, we purposely left out the maraschino cherry.

Butter-flavored cooking spray
1 pound lean, precooked smoked boneless pork chops or ham steaks
½ cup chopped onion
1 tablespoon balsamic vinegar
2 teaspoons concentrated chicken broth
½ cup water
Brown-sugar artificial sweetener (1 teaspoon equivalent)
½ cup diced fresh pineapple
½ teaspoon chili powder

1. In a large nonstick skillet, heat cooking spray over medium-high heat until hot but not smoking. Sauté pork for 2 minutes on one side, turn, and cook for 2 minutes on the other. Remove from pan and keep warm.
2. Add onion to pan and sauté for 2 minutes, or until soft.
3. Add balsamic vinegar, concentrated chicken broth, water, and sweetener, and stir to scrape up any browned bits. Stir in pineapple and chili powder, lower heat, and simmer for 3 minutes.
4. To serve, spoon pineapple sauce over smoked pork chops.

Makes 4 servings

SERVING GUIDELINES

▶ **FOR GASTRIC SLEEVE AND BYPASS:**
Week 1: Liquid diet.
Weeks 2–4: Puree 2 ounces cooked pork with 2 tablespoons sauce.
Weeks 5–7: Chop 2 ounces cooked pork and top with sauce.
Weeks 8+: Serve 2–4 ounces cooked pork topped with sauce.

▶ **FOR BPD-DS:**
Week 1: Liquid diet.
Weeks 2–3: Puree 2 ounces cooked pork with 2 tablespoons sauce.
Weeks 4+: Serve 3–4 ounces cooked pork topped with sauce.

▶ **FOR LAP-BAND:**
Week 1: Liquid diet.
Weeks 2–4: Puree 2 ounces cooked pork with 2 tablespoons sauce.
Weeks 5–7: Chop 2 ounces cooked pork and top with sauce.
Weeks 8+: Serve 2–4 ounces cooked pork topped with sauce.

▶ **FOR OTHERS:**
Serve 4 ounces cooked pork topped with sauce.

Calories: 165, **Protein:** 23 g, **Fat:** 5 g, **Carbohydrates:** 6 g, **Cholesterol:** 51 mg, **Fiber:** 1 g, **Sodium:** 1,651 mg

Spicy Orange Asian Pork Chops

Whether you like just a little heat or you really go for the burn, adjust the amount of garlic chili sauce to get just the degree of spice you want with these luscious chops.

Marinade:

¾ cup fresh orange juice
⅓ cup low-sodium soy sauce
1 teaspoon grated fresh ginger, or ½ teaspoon ground
1 to 3 teaspoons Asian chili sauce with garlic, or to taste
½ teaspoon sesame oil

4 bone-in ½-inch-thick pork chops
Canola cooking spray, canola oil, or other neutral-oil spray
1 large Vidalia or sweet onion, thinly sliced
1 pound string beans, trimmed
1 large carrot, peeled and cut into thin strips

1. *To make marinade:* Combine all marinade ingredients in a shallow pan big enough to hold pork chops. Add chops and marinate in refrigerator for 2 hours, turning once.
2. Preheat broiler and arrange rack to top position.
3. Reserving marinade, remove chops from marinade and pat dry.
4. Spray broiler pan with cooking spray and add chops. Broil chops for 5 minutes on each side.
5. While chops are broiling, spray a large lidded skillet with cooking spray and heat over high heat until hot but not smoking. Add onion, string beans, and carrots and cook, stirring often, for 2 minutes. Lower heat to medium. Pour in reserved marinade and cook, covered, for 4 to 6 minutes, or until beans and carrots are just tender. Taste sauce for spiciness. If needed, add more garlic chili sauce.
6. When chops are finished broiling, transfer from pan to individual plates. Spoon sauce and vegetables over and around them.

Makes 4 servings

SERVING GUIDELINES

➤ **FOR GASTRIC SLEEVE AND BYPASS:**
Week 1: Liquid diet.
Weeks 2–7: Puree 2 ounces cooked pork with 2 tablespoons veggies and sauce.
Weeks 8+: Serve 2–4 ounces cooked pork with 2 tablespoons veggies and sauce.

➤ **FOR BPD-DS:**
Week 1: Liquid diet.
Weeks 2–7: Puree 2 ounces cooked pork with 2 tablespoons veggies and sauce.
Weeks 8+: Serve 2–4 ounces cooked pork with 2 tablespoons veggies and sauce.

➤ **FOR LAP-BAND:**
Week 1: Liquid diet.
Weeks 2–7: Puree 2 ounces cooked pork with 2 tablespoons veggies and sauce.
Weeks 8+: Serve 2–4 ounces cooked pork with 2 tablespoons veggies and sauce.

➤ **FOR OTHERS:**
Serve 4 ounces cooked pork with veggies and sauce.

Calories: 238, **Protein:** 27 g, **Fat:** 5 g, **Carbohydrates:** 19 g, **Cholesterol:** 55 mg, **Fiber:** 6 g, **Sodium:** 923 mg

Beef Bordelaise

This dish is so good that I often double it and freeze half or serve it two days in a row. The secret ingredient? The orange peel. It really adds a bit of zing.

Olive oil cooking spray
1 pound lean beef round, trimmed and
  cut into 1-inch cubes
1½ cups chopped onion
2 large garlic cloves, chopped
½ cup dry red wine
½ cup fat-free, low-sodium beef broth
1 cup chopped tomato
1 (6-ounce) can tomato juice
1 (3 x 1-inch) piece orange peel
1 teaspoon Worcestershire sauce
1 teaspoon chopped fresh rosemary,
  or ½ teaspoon dried
½ pound peeled baby carrots

1. In a heavy pot, heat cooking spray over medium-high heat until hot but not smoking. Brown beef on all sides and transfer to a bowl.
2. Discard any fat accumulated in pot. Add onion and garlic to pot and cook over medium heat, stirring, for 2 minutes, or until golden.
3. Add wine, broth, tomato, tomato juice, orange peel, Worcestershire, and rosemary to pot and bring to a boil. Add back to pot beef and any meat juices that have accumulated.
4. Cover and lower heat; simmer for 30 minutes.
5. Stir in carrots, cover, and simmer for 1½ hours.
6. Uncover, increase heat to medium-high, and cook for 15 minutes, or until liquid in pot reduces and is slightly thickened.

Makes 4 servings
➤ **Hint:** This recipe can be made up to 3 days ahead and refrigerated.

SERVING GUIDELINES

➤ **FOR GASTRIC SLEEVE AND BYPASS:**
  Week 1: Liquid diet.
  Weeks 2–4: Puree 2 ounces cooked beef with 2 tablespoons vegetables and sauce.
  Weeks 5–7: Chop 2 ounces cooked beef and top with vegetables and sauce.
  Weeks 8+: Serve 2–4 ounces cooked beef topped with vegetables and sauce.

➤ **FOR BPD-DS:**
  Week 1: Liquid diet.
  Weeks 2–3: Puree 2–3 ounces cooked beef with 2 tablespoons vegetables and sauce.
  Weeks 4+: Serve 3–4 ounces cooked beef topped with vegetables and sauce.

➤ **FOR LAP-BAND:**
  Week 1: Liquid diet.
  Weeks 2–4: Puree 2 ounces cooked beef with 2 tablespoons vegetables and sauce.
  Weeks 5–7: Chop 2 ounces cooked beef and top with vegetables and sauce.
  Weeks 8+: Serve 2–4 ounces cooked beef topped with vegetables and sauce.

➤ **FOR OTHERS:**
  Serve 4 ounces cooked beef topped with vegetables and sauce.

Calories: 244, **Protein:** 27 g, **Fat:** 4 g, **Carbohydrates:** 16 g, **Cholesterol:** 60 mg, **Fiber:** 3 g, **Sodium:** 133 mg

Mom's Pot Roast

Yes, this really is my mother's pot roast recipe. The coffee, while not an expected ingredient, makes this pot roast intensely flavorful.

Olive oil cooking spray
2 pounds lean beef brisket
1½ cups coarsely chopped onion
2 garlic cloves, minced
2 tablespoons sweet paprika
1 (14.5-ounce) can low-sodium beef broth
1 cup strong brewed coffee
1 cup water
2 tablespoons concentrated beef broth
2 bay leaves
1 ounce dried mushrooms
1½ cups coarsely chopped carrot
¾ pound green beans, ends trimmed
Salt and pepper to taste

1. In a 4- to 5-quart nonstick Dutch oven, heat cooking spray over medium-high heat until hot but not smoking. Place meat in Dutch oven and brown on both sides, about 5 minutes. Remove meat from pot and pour off accumulated fat.
2. Place onion, garlic, and paprika in pot, stir, cover, and cook over medium heat for 5 to 7 minutes, or until onion is softened.
3. Add meat back to pot on top of onion mixture and pour in beef broth, coffee, and water. Stir in concentrated beef broth, and bring to a boil. Then, add bay leaves, mushrooms, and carrot, lower heat to a simmer, cover, and cook for 1½ hours.
4. Remove meat from pot and slice thinly on diagonal.
5. Add meat back to pot, place green beans on top, cover, and cook for another 30 minutes. Add salt and pepper to taste.

Makes 8 servings

► **Cooking Tip:** This dish can be made a day ahead and refrigerated until you're ready to serve. Just remember to skim off the fat before reheating.

SERVING GUIDELINES

► **FOR GATRIC SLEEVE AND BYPASS:**
  Week 1: Liquid diet.
  Weeks 2–4: Puree 2 ounces cooked beef with 2 tablespoons vegetables and sauce.
  Weeks 5–7: Chop 2 ounces cooked beef and top with vegetables and sauce.
  Weeks 8+: Serve 2–4 ounces cooked beef with vegetables and sauce.

► **FOR BPD-DS:**
  Week 1: Liquid diet.
  Weeks 2–3: Puree 2 ounces cooked beef with 2 tablespoons vegetables and sauce.
  Weeks 4+: Serve 2–4 ounces cooked beef with vegetables and sauce.

► **FOR LAP-BAND:**
  Week 1: Liquid diet.
  Weeks 2–4: Puree 2 ounces cooked beef with 2 tablespoons vegetables and sauce.
  Weeks 5–7: Chop 2 ounces cooked beef and top with vegetables and sauce.
  Weeks 8+: Serve 2–4 ounces cooked beef with vegetables and sauce.

► **FOR OTHERS:**
  Serve 4 ounces of cooked beef with vegetables and sauce.

Calories: 231, **Protein:** 27 g, **Fat:** 9 g, **Carbohydrates:** 11 g, **Cholesterol:** 70 mg, **Fiber:** 3 g, **Sodium:** 681 mg

Beef Stroganoff

Everything about this recipe is authentic to the original Russian dish, except we left out all the fat.

Butter-flavored cooking spray
2 garlic cloves, minced
1 pound lean eye round, cut into
  1-inch cubes
1 (6-ounce) can tomato sauce
½ cup dry red wine
1 cup sliced fresh mushrooms
1 bay leaf
½ cup fat-free sour cream
Salt and pepper to taste

1. Coat bottom of large nonstick lidded skillet with cooking spray and heat over medium-high heat until hot. Sauté garlic for 1 minute until soft. Add meat and brown, stirring, for 3 minutes.
2. Add tomato sauce, wine, mushrooms, and bay leaf and lower heat. Simmer, covered, over low heat for 1½ hours.
3. Turn off heat and stir in sour cream. Add salt and pepper to taste.

Makes 4 servings

SERVING GUIDELINES

▶ **FOR GASTRIC SLEEVE AND BYPASS:**
   Week 1: Liquid diet.
   Weeks 2–4: Puree 2 ounces cooked meat with 2 tablespoons sauce.
   Weeks 5–7: Chop 2 ounces cooked meat and top with sauce.
   Weeks 8+: Serve 2–4 ounces cooked meat with sauce.

▶ **FOR BPD-DS:**
   Week 1: Liquid diet.
   Weeks 2–3: Puree 2 ounces cooked meat with 2 tablespoons sauce.
   Weeks 4+: Serve 3–4 ounces cooked meat with sauce.

▶ **FOR LAP-BAND:**
   Week 1: Liquid diet.
   Weeks 2–4: Puree 2 ounces cooked meat with 2 tablespoons sauce.
   Weeks 5–7: Chop 2 ounces cooked meat and top with sauce.
   Weeks 8+: Serve 2–4 ounces cooked meat with sauce.

▶ **FOR OTHERS:**
   Serve 4 ounces cooked meat with sauce.

Calories: 229, **Protein:** 27 g, **Fat:** 4 g, **Carbohydrates:** 10 g, **Cholesterol:** 65 mg, **Fiber:** 1 g, **Sodium:** 254 mg

Flank Steak Basquaise

Recipes from the Basque section of Spain often use a savory mixture of bell pepper, onion, and tomato. We added wine and mushrooms just 'cause we like them.

Olive oil cooking spray
1 pound lean flank steak
½ cup chopped onion
2 garlic cloves, chopped
½ cup seeded and chopped red
    bell pepper
½ pound sliced fresh mushrooms
½ cup dry red wine
½ cup chopped plum tomatoes
2 teaspoons concentrated beef broth
Salt and pepper to taste

1. Preheat broiler and arrange rack to top position.
2. Spray broiler pan with cooking spray and place flank steak on top. With a sharp knife, score top of steak so it won't curl. Broil for 3 to 5 minutes on each side, or until medium rare.
3. While steak is broiling, heat cooking spray in a medium nonstick skillet over medium-high heat until it's hot but not smoking. Sauté onion and garlic for 3 minutes, or until lightly browned.
4. Add bell pepper and mushrooms and cook, covered, for 3 to 5 minutes, or until soft. Add wine, tomatoes, and beef broth concentrate and cook, stirring occasionally, until liquid is reduced by half.
5. Slice steak very thinly on diagonal. Add salt and pepper to taste. Spoon vegetable-wine sauce on top.

Makes 4 servings

SERVING GUIDELINES

▶ **FOR GASTRIC SLEEVE AND BYPASS:**
   Week 1: Liquid diet.
   Weeks 2–4: Puree 2 ounces cooked meat with 2 tablespoons sauce.
   Weeks 5–7: Chop 2 ounces cooked meat and top with sauce.
   Weeks 8+: Serve 2–4 ounces cooked meat with sauce.

▶ **FOR BPD-DS:**
   Week 1: Liquid diet.
   Weeks 2–3: Puree 2 ounces cooked meat with 2 tablespoons sauce.
   Weeks 4+: Serve 3–4 ounces cooked meat with sauce.

▶ **FOR LAP-BAND:**
   Week 1: Liquid diet.
   Weeks 2–4: Puree 2 ounces cooked meat with 2 tablespoons sauce.
   Weeks 5–7: Chop 2 ounces cooked meat and top with sauce.
   Weeks 8+: Serve 2–4 ounces cooked meat with sauce.

▶ **FOR OTHERS:**
   Serve 4 ounces cooked meat with sauce.

Calories: 230, **Protein:** 24 g, **Fat:** 10 g, **Carbohydrates:** 9 g, **Cholesterol:** 65 mg, **Fiber:** 2 g, **Sodium:** 292 mg

London Broil with Horseradish Cream

The British traditionally serve beef with horseradish. Here is a flavorful variation on that classic theme.

1 pound lean London broil (top round or flank steak)
1½ teaspoons garlic powder
1 tablespoon lemon-pepper
½ cup fat-free sour cream
1 tablespoon concentrated beef broth
2 tablespoons prepared horseradish

1. Preheat broiler and arrange rack to top position.
2. With a sharp knife, score top of London broil to keep it from curling. Sprinkle with garlic powder and lemon-pepper.
3. Place in nonstick broiling pan and broil for 4 minutes on each side for medium rare.
4. While steak is broiling, combine sour cream, concentrated beef broth, and horseradish in a small bowl.
5. Slice steak thinly on diagonal, pour sauce over it, and serve.

Makes 4 servings

SERVING GUIDELINES

► **FOR GASTRIC SLEEVE AND BYPASS:**
Week 1: Liquid diet.
Weeks 2–4: Puree 2 ounces cooked meat with 2 tablespoons sauce.
Weeks 5–7: Chop 2 ounces cooked meat and top with sauce.
Weeks 8+: Serve 2–4 ounces cooked meat with sauce.

► **FOR BPD-DS:**
Week 1: Liquid diet.
Weeks 2–3: Puree 2 ounces cooked meat with 2 tablespoons sauce.
Weeks 4+: Serve 3–4 ounces cooked meat with sauce.

► **FOR LAP-BAND:**
Week 1: Liquid diet.
Weeks 2–4: Puree 2 ounces cooked meat with 2 tablespoons sauce.
Weeks 5–7: Chop 2 ounces cooked meat and top with sauce.
Weeks 8+: Serve 2–4 ounces cooked meat with sauce.

► **FOR OTHERS:**
Serve 4 ounces cooked meat with sauce.

Calories: 182, **Protein:** 28 g, **Fat:** 5 g, **Carbohydrates:** 8 g, **Cholesterol:** 65 mg, **Fiber:** 0 g, **Sodium:** 723 mg

Soy-Mustard Glazed Beef

All the ingredients in this dish shouldn't work together, but they do. The glaze creates a seared crust on the meat, while the creamy sauce complements it perfectly.

Glaze:

⅓ cup light soy sauce

2 tablespoons Dijon mustard

1 tablespoon fresh lemon juice

4 garlic cloves, quartered

1½ teaspoons minced fresh ginger

½ teaspoon dried thyme

½ teaspoon freshly ground black pepper

½ teaspoon fresh rosemary

Olive oil cooking spray

1 pound lean London broil (lean top round or flank steak)

½ cup fat-free sour cream

1 tablespoon concentrated beef broth

¼ teaspoon sesame oil

1. *To make glaze:* In a mini-processor or blender, combine glaze ingredients and process until smooth. Reserve 2 tablespoons of glaze mixture to make sauce.
2. Preheat broiler and arrange rack to top position. Spray a broiling pan with cooking spray.
3. Brush top of steak with glaze mixture, place on broiling pan and broil for 3 to 4 minutes. Turn steak, brush other side with glaze, and broil for 3 to 4 minutes longer for medium rare.
4. In a small bowl, combine reserved glaze with sour cream, concentrated beef broth, and sesame oil.
5. Slice steak thinly on diagonal, pour sauce over it, and serve.

Makes 4 servings

SERVING GUIDELINES

► **FOR GASTRIC SLEEVE AND BYPASS:**
Week 1: Liquid diet.
Weeks 2–4: Puree 2 ounces cooked meat with 2 tablespoons sauce.
Weeks 5–7: Chop 2 ounces cooked meat and top with sauce.
Weeks 8+: Serve 2–4 ounces cooked meat with sauce.

► **FOR BPD-DS:**
Week 1: Liquid diet.
Weeks 2–3: Puree 2 ounces cooked meat with 2 tablespoons sauce.
Weeks 4+: Serve 3–4 ounces cooked meat with sauce.

► **FOR LAP-BAND:**
Week 1: Liquid diet.
Weeks 2–4: Puree 2 ounces cooked meat with 2 tablespoons sauce.
Weeks 5–7: Chop 2 ounces cooked meat and top with sauce.
Weeks 8+: Serve 2–4 ounces cooked meat with sauce.

► **FOR OTHERS:**
Serve 4 ounces cooked meat with sauce.

Calories: 249, **Protein:** 27 g, **Fat:** 10 g, **Carbohydrates:** 12 g, **Cholesterol:** 70 mg, **Fiber:** 0 g, **Sodium:** 1,188 mg

Savory Onion and Mushroom Burgers

You won't miss the hamburger buns when you taste how delectable these burgers are.

Olive oil cooking spray
1 large sweet onion, sliced thinly and
    separated into rings (about 1½ cups)
2 cups sliced fresh mushrooms
1 tablespoon sweet paprika
¼ teaspoon cayenne pepper
½ teaspoon dried thyme
¼ teaspoon freshly ground black pepper
1 pound lean ground round
2 tablespoons balsamic vinegar
2 tablespoons concentrated beef broth
½ cup water
2 tablespoons prepared horseradish

1. Coat bottom of a medium nonstick skillet with cooking spray. Sauté onion rings over medium-high heat for 5 minutes, or until slightly browned.

2. Add mushrooms and cover, lower heat to medium, and cook for 5 minutes, or until mushrooms give up their liquid. Remove onion-mushroom mixture from pan and set aside.

3. While onion-mushroom mixture is cooking, mix together paprika, cayenne, thyme, and black pepper in a shallow bowl.

4. Divide and shape meat into four patties; dredge patties on both sides in spice mixture.

5. Re-spray empty pan with cooking spray and sauté patties over medium-high heat on one side for 4 minutes. Flip patties over, cover pan, and cook for 3 to 4 more minutes, or until medium-rare. Remove burgers from pan and discard any accumulated fat.

6. Deglaze pan with balsamic vinegar, scraping up any browned bits. Add concentrated broth, water, and horseradish, bring to a simmer, and add onion-mushroom mixture back to pan.

7. Simmer, uncovered, stirring occasionally, for 3 minutes, or until slightly reduced.

Makes 4 servings

SERVING GUIDELINES

- **FOR GASTRIC SLEEVE AND BYPASS:**
  Week 1: Liquid diet.
  Weeks 2–4: Puree ½ cooked burger (2 ounces) with 2 tablespoons onion-mushroom sauce.
  Weeks 5–7+: Serve ½–1 cooked burger topped with onion-mushroom sauce.
  Weeks 8+: Serve ½–1 cooked burger topped with 2 tablespoons onion-mushroom sauce.

- **FOR BPD-DS:**
  Week 1: Liquid diet.
  Weeks 2–3: Puree ½ cooked burger (2 ounces) with 2 tablespoons onion-mushroom sauce.
  Weeks 4+: Serve ½–1 cooked burger topped with onion-mushroom sauce.

- **FOR LAP-BAND:**
  Week 1: Liquid diet.
  Weeks 2–4: Puree ½ cooked burger (2 ounces) with 2 tablespoons onion-mushroom sauce.
  Weeks 5–7+: Serve ½–1 cooked burger topped with onion-mushroom sauce.
  Weeks 8+: Serve ½–1 cooked burger topped with 2 tablespoons onion-mushroom sauce.

- **FOR OTHERS:**
  Serve 1 cooked burger topped with onion-mushroom sauce.

Calories: 203, **Protein:** 26 g, **Fat:** 7 g, **Carbohydrates:** 11 g, **Cholesterol:** 62 mg, **Fiber:** 2 g, **Sodium:** 958 mg

Pan-Grilled Burgers with
Blue Cheese–Horseradish Cream

I have learned to love burgers without buns, especially if they are topped with something as luscious as this creamy, spicy, tangy sauce.

1 pound lean ground beef

2 tablespoons steak or beef rub (I use Penzeys English Prime Rib Rub)

Butter-flavored cooking spray

½ cup reduced-fat sour cream

1 tablespoon prepared horseradish

2 teaspoons Bovrite or other condensed beef broth

1 tablespoon crumbled blue cheese

1. Divide and shape meat into four 1-inch-thick patties. Sprinkle steak rub on both sides of patties and press so that seasoning sticks to meat.

2. Heat a heavy skillet over medium-high heat until very hot and spray with cooking spray. Cook patties for 4 minutes on one side, flip, and cook for 4 minutes on other side.

3. While burgers are cooking, mix sour cream, horseradish, and condensed beef broth in small bowl. Add blue cheese and stir until combined.

Makes 4 servings

SERVING GUIDELINES

► **FOR GASTRIC SLEEVE AND BYPASS:**
Week 1: Liquid diet.
Weeks 2–3: Puree ½ cooked burger with 2 tablespoons sauce.
Weeks 4–7: Chop ½ cooked burger and top with 2 tablespoons sauce.
Weeks 8+: Serve ½–1 cooked burger topped with 2 tablespoons sauce.

► **FOR BPD-DS:**
Week 1: Liquid diet.
Weeks 2–3: Puree ½ cooked burger with 2 tablespoons sauce.
Weeks 4+: Serve ½–1 cooked burger topped with 2 tablespoons sauce.

► **FOR LAP-BAND:**
Week 1: Liquid diet.
Weeks 2–3: Puree ½ cooked burger with 2 tablespoons sauce.
Weeks 4–7: Chop ½ cooked burger and top with 2 tablespoons sauce.
Weeks 8+: Serve ½–1 cooked burger topped with 2 tablespoons sauce.

► **FOR OTHERS:**
Serve 1 cooked burger topped with sauce.

Calories: 167, **Protein:** 25 g, **Fat:** 5 g, **Carbohydrates:** 5 g, **Cholesterol:** 71 mg, **Fiber:** 0 g, **Sodium:** 383 mg

Mom's Meatloaf

You know how everyone adds ketchup to a meatloaf recipe? Not my mother. She used a small can of tomato juice. The result? A really moist meatloaf.

1 pound lean ground beef, preferably ground round
1 large egg, lightly beaten
1 (5.4-ounce) can tomato juice
2 tablespoons concentrated beef broth
½ cup minced onion
2 tablespoons dried parsley
1 teaspoon garlic powder
1 teaspoon steak rub (I use Penzeys English Prime Rib Rub)
¼ cup gluten-free unseasoned panko (crispy Japanese-style bread crumbs)
Butter-flavored cooking spray

1. Preheat oven to 350°F.
2. In a large bowl, using your hands, break up ground beef.
3. In a smaller bowl, combine egg, tomato juice, condensed beef broth, onion, parsley, garlic, and steak rub.
4. Pour egg–tomato juice mixture into beef and mix thoroughly.
5. Add panko to beef mixture and knead it until well blended.
6. Coat a baking pan with cooking spray. Mound meat mixture in center of pan to form a loaf and bake for 1 hour.

Makes 4 servings

► **Note:** For those who automatically put ketchup on top of their meatloaf (like my husband), try our Shallot-Horseradish Sauce (page 190) or Sauce Basquaise (page 195) instead.

SERVING GUIDELINES

► **FOR GASTRIC SLEEVE AND BYPASS:**
  Week 1: Liquid diet.
  Weeks 2–3: Puree 2 ounces cooked meatloaf.
  Weeks 4–7: Chop 2 ounces cooked meatloaf.
  Weeks 8+: Serve 2–4 ounces cooked meatloaf.

► **FOR BPD-DS:**
  Week 1: Liquid diet.
  Weeks 2–3: Puree 2 ounces cooked meatloaf.
  Weeks 4–7: Chop 2 ounces cooked meatloaf.
  Weeks 8+: Serve 2–4 ounces cooked meatloaf.

► **FOR LAP-BAND:**
  Week 1: Liquid diet.
  Weeks 2–3: Puree 2 ounces cooked meatloaf.
  Weeks 4–7: Chop 2 ounces cooked meatloaf.
  Weeks 8+: Serve 2–4 ounces cooked meatloaf.

► **FOR OTHERS:**
  Serve 4 ounces cooked meatloaf.

Calories: 203, **Protein:** 27 g, **Fat:** 5 g, **Carbohydrates:** 12 g, **Cholesterol:** 112 mg, **Fiber:** 1 g, **Sodium:** 345 mg

Asian Stir-fry

This is a classic stir-fry but feel free to change it up by using chicken, pork, shrimp, or tofu instead of beef and a variety of different veggies. If you like, the stir-fry can be served over cauliflower rice.

Sauce:

⅓ cup low-sodium soy sauce

2 tablespoons rice vinegar

¼ cup dry sherry (I use cooking sherry; optional)

1 teaspoon grated or minced fresh ginger, or ½ teaspoon ground

1 teaspoon sesame oil

2 packets artificial sweetener (Splenda or Truvia)

Canola or other neutral-flavored cooking spray

1 pound lean beef, sliced thinly

1 large sweet onion, peeled, cut in half, and sliced into ¼-inch slices

1 clove garlic, minced

2 scallions or green onions (white and green parts), sliced into ¼-inch slices

1 red, yellow, or orange bell pepper, seeded and cut into ¼-inch slices

4 large white mushrooms, sliced

1 medium zucchini, cut into ¼ inch rounds

½ pound snow peas or sugar snap peas, stringed, cut in half diagonally

½ head bok choy or 2 heads baby bok choy, washed thoroughly, then sliced on the diagonal into ½-inch slices

1. *To make sauce:* In a saucepan, combine all sauce ingredients and bring to a simmer.
2. Spray cooking spray in wok or large lidded skillet, then heat over medium-high heat until it shimmers. Add sliced beef and stir-fry for 2 minutes, or until barely browned. Remove beef from pan and keep warm.
3. Wipe pan, re-spray, and heat until shimmering. Add onion and garlic and cook, stirring, for about 4 minutes, or until translucent, but do not brown.
4. Stir in scallions, peppers, mushrooms, and zucchini. Add sauce and cook, stirring, for 3 to 4 minutes.
5. Stir in peas and bok choy, cover, and steam for 2 minutes.
6. Stir beef back into pan and cook for 2 minutes, or until heated through.

Makes 4 servings

SERVING GUIDELINES

➤ **FOR GASTRIC SLEEVE AND BYPASS:**
Week 1: Liquid diet.
Weeks 2–4: Puree 2 ounces cooked beef and vegetables with 2 tablespoons sauce.
Weeks 5–7: Chop 2 ounces cooked beef and vegetables and top with 2 tablespoons sauce.
Weeks 8+: Serve 2–4 ounces cooked beef topped with sauce and vegetables.

➤ **FOR BPD-DS:**
Week 1: Liquid diet.
Weeks 1–3: Puree 2–3 ounces cooked beef and vegetables with 2 tablespoons sauce.
Weeks 4+: Serve 3–4 ounces cooked beef and vegetables with 2 tablespoons sauce.

➤ **FOR LAP-BAND:**
Week 1: Liquid diet.
Weeks 2–4: Puree 2 ounces cooked beef and vegetables with 2 tablespoons sauce.
Weeks 5–7: Chop 2 ounces cooked beef and vegetables and top with 2 tablespoons sauce.
Weeks 8+: Serve 2–4 ounces cooked beef topped with sauce and vegetables.

➤ **FOR OTHERS:**
Serve 4 ounces cooked beef with 1 cup vegetables and sauce.

Calories: 334, **Protein:** 27 g, **Fat:** 12 g, **Carbohydrates:** 23 g, **Cholesterol:** 75 mg, **Fiber:** 4 g, **Sodium:** 899 mg

Tuscan Veal Stew

This is a light, brightly spiced stew that can be made a day or two ahead and kept in the refrigerator. I usually save this recipe for "Sunday cooking."

1 (14.5-ounce) can low-sodium chicken broth
1 cup (8 whole) sun-dried tomatoes (not oil-packed), quartered
Olive oil cooking spray
1 pound lean veal, cut into 1-inch cubes
½ cup white wine
1 cup sliced fresh mushrooms
½ cup plain, fat-free yogurt
1 small fresh red or green serrano or jalapeño pepper, seeded and sliced in half
1 teaspoon fresh rosemary
Salt and pepper to taste

1. In shallow glass bowl, heat chicken broth in microwave on HIGH for 45 seconds or bring broth to boil in a small saucepan. Soak sun-dried tomatoes in warm broth for 15 minutes.

2. Coat bottom of 4- to 5-quart nonstick pot with cooking spray and heat over medium-high heat until hot but not smoking. Brown veal for 3 minutes, turning occasionally, until golden (if necessary, brown in 2 batches). Transfer to a bowl.

3. Deglaze pot with wine, scraping up any browned bits. Add veal and any meat juices that have accumulated back to pot. Add sun-dried tomatoes and broth, mushrooms, yogurt, chile pepper, and rosemary.

4. Lower heat to low and simmer, covered, stirring occasionally, for about 1¼ hours, or until veal is tender.

5. Discard chile pepper and add salt and pepper to taste.

Makes 4 servings

SERVING GUIDELINES

► **FOR GASTRIC SLEEVE AND BYPASS:**
Week 1: Liquid diet.
Weeks 2–4: Puree 2 ounces cooked veal with 2 tablespoons vegetables and sauce.
Weeks 5–7: Chop 2 ounces cooked veal and top with vegetables and sauce.
Weeks 8+: Serve 2–4 ounces cooked veal topped with vegetables and sauce.

► **FOR BPD-DS:**
Week 1: Liquid diet.
Weeks 2–3: Puree 2 ounces cooked veal with 2 tablespoons vegetables and sauce.
Weeks 4+: Serve 3–4 ounces cooked veal topped with vegetables and sauce.

► **FOR LAP-BAND:**
Week 1: Liquid diet.
Weeks 2–4: Puree 2 ounces cooked veal with 2 tablespoons vegetables and sauce.
Weeks 5–7: Chop 2 ounces cooked veal and top with vegetables and sauce.
Weeks 8+: Serve 2–4 ounces cooked veal topped with vegetables and sauce.

► **FOR OTHERS:**
Serve 4 ounces cooked veal topped with vegetables and sauce.

Calories: 189, **Protein:** 27 g, **Fat:** 4 g, **Carbohydrates:** 8 g, **Cholesterol:** 95 mg, **Fiber:** 1 g, **Sodium:** 525 mg

Greek Lamb Burgers with Yogurt-Mint Sauce

Instead of grilled lamb, we've taken a classic recipe and turned it into burgers so you can enjoy this dish even on a weeknight.

Burgers:

3 or 4 scallions (white and light green parts only), chopped (about ¾ cup)
1 pound lean ground lamb
1 teaspoon ground cumin
1 teaspoon ground coriander
Salt and pepper to taste
Olive oil cooking spray

Yogurt-Mint Sauce
(makes approximately 1 cup):

½ teaspoon fresh lemon zest
½ cup fresh mint leaves
1 small garlic clove, quartered
¾ cup plain, fat-free yogurt
1 teaspoon ground cumin
1 tablespoon fresh lemon juice
2 teaspoons concentrated chicken broth

1. Mix scallions, lamb, and seasonings in bowl so they are well blended. Divide and form into four patties.
2. In a medium nonstick skillet, heat cooking spray over medium-high heat until hot but not smoking. Place patties in skillet and cook for 4 minutes, then turn over and cook for 4 minutes more for medium rare.
3. While meat is cooking, combine lemon zest, mint, and garlic in mini-processor or chopper and finely chop.
4. In a medium-size bowl, mix yogurt, cumin, lemon juice, and concentrated chicken broth. Add chopped mint mixture and mix well.
5. Remove burgers from skillet and drain on paper towels. Serve burgers with sauce spooned on top.

Makes 4 servings

SERVING GUIDELINES

► **FOR GASTRIC SLEEVE AND BYPASS:**
  Week 1: Liquid diet.
  Weeks 2–4: Puree ½ cooked burger (2 ounces)
    with 2 tablespoons sauce.
  Weeks 5+: Serve ½–1 cooked burger topped with
    2 tablespoons sauce.

► **FOR BPD-DS:**
  Week 1: Liquid diet.
  Weeks 2–3: Puree ½ cooked burger (2 ounces)
    with 2 tablespoons sauce.
  Weeks 4+: Serve ½–1 cooked burger topped with
    2 tablespoons sauce.

► **FOR LAP-BAND:**
  Week 1: Liquid diet.
  Weeks 2–4: Puree ½ cooked burger (2 ounces)
    with 2 tablespoons sauce.
  Weeks 5+: Serve ½–1 cooked burger topped with
    2 tablespoons sauce.

► **FOR OTHERS:**
  Serve 1 cooked burger topped with sauce.

Burgers:

Calories: 331, **Protein:** 19 g, **Fat:** 27 g, **Carbohydrates:** 2 g, **Cholesterol:** 83 mg, **Fiber:** 1 g, **Sodium:** 71 mg

Yogurt-Mint Sauce (2 tablespoons):

Calories: 15, **Protein:** 1 g, **Fat:** 0 g, **Carbohydrates:** 3 g, **Cholesterol:** 0 mg, **Fiber:** 1 g, **Sodium:** 52 mg

Moussaka

Here is a lighter version of this classic Greek dish. We substituted ground turkey for half of the ground lamb and used skim milk for the custard, but it still tastes authentic. It is kind of labor intensive, so why not make it for Sunday dinner?

1 large eggplant (about 1½ pounds)
½ teaspoon salt
Canola cooking spray
½ pound lean ground lamb
½ pound lean ground turkey
1 cup diced onion
1 garlic clove, minced
¼ pound (4 to 5 large) mushrooms,
    coarsely chopped
¼ cup red wine
1 (8-ounce) can tomato sauce
1 tablespoon dried parsley flakes
1 tablespoon chopped fresh oregano,
    or 1½ teaspoons dried
¼ teaspoon ground cinnamon
Salt and pepper to taste

Custard Topping:
1½ cups skim milk
½ cup egg substitute
½ cup plus 2 tablespoons grated
    Parmesan cheese

1. Preheat oven to 400°F.
2. Cut ends off eggplant and slice horizontally into ¼-inch-thick slices. Line a colander with eggplant slices, sprinkle with salt, and let drain for 30 minutes.
3. Coat a large nonstick skillet with cooking spray and cook lamb and turkey over medium heat, stirring vigorously to mix well and break up lumps. Brown for about 5 minutes, then drain off fat.
4. Add onion, garlic, and mushrooms and cook over medium heat about 3 minutes. Add wine, tomato sauce, and seasonings, stir, and cook for 2 more minutes.
5. *To make custard:* While eggplant is draining, whisk together milk, egg substitute, and ½ cup Parmesan cheese in a medium saucepan. Stirring constantly, simmer over low heat for 5 to 7 minutes, or until slightly thickened and reduced by one third. Remove from heat and set aside.
6. *To assemble:* Lightly coat a baking pan with cooking spray.
7. Rinse eggplant and pat dry. Layer half of eggplant slices on bottom and top with half of lamb-turkey mixture. Layer with rest of eggplant and top with remaining lamb-turkey. Pour custard over top and sprinkle it with remaining 2 tablespoons grated Parmesan cheese.
8. Bake for 45 minutes to 1 hour, or until golden.

Makes 4 servings

SERVING GUIDELINES

► **FOR GASTRIC SLEEVE AND BYPASS:**
  Week 1: Liquid diet.
  Weeks 2–4: Puree ½ cup moussaka until smooth.
  Weeks 5+: Serve ½ cup moussaka as is.

► **FOR BPD-DS:**
  Week 1: Liquid diet.
  Weeks 2–3: Puree ½ cup moussaka.
  Weeks 4+: Serve ½–1 cup moussaka as is.

► **FOR LAP-BAND:**
  Week 1: Liquid diet.
  Weeks 2–4: Puree ½ cup moussaka.
  Weeks 5+: Serve ½ cup moussaka as is.

► **FOR OTHERS:**
  Serve 1 cup moussaka as is.

Moussaka:

Calories: 318, **Protein:** 27 g, **Fat:** 15 g, **Carbohydrates:** 19 g, **Cholesterol:** 69 mg, **Fiber:** 6 g, **Sodium:** 345 mg

Custard Topping:

Calories: 105, **Protein:** 11 g, **Fat:** 5 g, **Carbohydrates:** 8 g, **Cholesterol:** 12 mg, **Fiber:** 0 g, **Sodium:** 335 mg

Moussaka with Custard Topping:

Calories: 422, **Protein:** 39 g, **Fat:** 20 g, **Carbohydrates:** 27 g, **Cholesterol:** 81 mg, **Fiber:** 6 g, **Sodium:** 680 mg

Peppercorn and Mustard Crusted Lamb Chops

Mustard, garlic, and pepper just seem to go well with lamb. Then, mellow the heat out with a creamy sauce—yum!

2 tablespoons mixed or black whole peppercorns, coarsely ground
2 tablespoons whole-grain mustard
3 tablespoons bottled minced roasted garlic
4 lamb chops, ½ inch thick, well trimmed of fat
Olive oil cooking spray
1 cup low-sodium beef broth
2 tablespoons fresh lemon juice
½ teaspoon dried mint
½ cup reduced-fat sour cream

1. Preheat oven to 375°F.
2. Combine ground peppercorns, mustard, and garlic to form a paste. Spread all over chops.
3. Spray a baking dish with olive oil spray. Place chops in dish and bake for 15 to 17 minutes.
4. While chops are baking, combine broth, lemon juice, and mint in a small saucepan and bring to a boil, then lower heat and simmer for about 15 minutes.
5. Turn off heat. Add sour cream to broth mixture and stir until smooth. Serve with lamb chops.

Makes 4 servings

SERVING GUIDELINES

► **FOR GASTRIC SLEEVE AND BYPASS:**
   Week 1: Liquid diet.
   Weeks 2–7: Puree 2 ounces cooked lamb with 2 tablespoons sauce.
   Weeks 8+: Serve 2–4 ounces cooked lamb with 2 tablespoons sauce.

► **FOR BPD-DS:**
   Week 1: Liquid diet.
   Weeks 2–7: Puree 2 ounces cooked lamb with 2 tablespoons sauce.
   Weeks 8+: Serve 2–4 ounces cooked lamb with 2 tablespoons sauce.

► **FOR LAP-BAND:**
   Week 1: Liquid diet.
   Weeks 2–7: Puree 2 ounces cooked lamb with 2 tablespoons sauce.
   Weeks 8+: Serve 2–4 ounces cooked lamb with 2 tablespoons sauce.

► **FOR OTHERS:**
   Serve 4 ounces cooked lamb with sauce.

Calories: 211, **Protein:** 29 g, **Fat:** 7 g, **Carbohydrates:** 4 g, **Cholesterol:** 10 mg, **Fiber:** 0 g, **Sodium:** 290 mg

Spiced Lamb Chops

This is kinda Greek, sorta Middle Eastern, but totally terrific. The spices combined with the tang of yogurt and lime really marry well with lamb.

2 garlic cloves, finely minced
¼ teaspoon ground cumin
¼ teaspoon ground cardamom
2 tablespoons water
1 teaspoon concentrated chicken broth
1 pound shoulder lamb chops (about 4),
    ½ inch thick, well trimmed of fat
Olive oil cooking spray
¾ cup plain, fat-free yogurt
1 tablespoon fresh lime juice
Salt and pepper to taste

1. In a shallow dish, stir together garlic, cumin, cardamom, water, and concentrated chicken broth. Dip lamb chops in mixture, turning once to coat well. Cover with foil and marinate at room temperature for 15 minutes.

2. Coat a large nonstick skillet with cooking spray and heat over medium-high heat until hot but not smoking. Reserving marinade, remove lamb chops from marinade. Cook lamb chops for about 3 minutes on each side for medium rare. Transfer lamb to a platter and keep warm.

3. Add yogurt and lime juice to reserved marinade, pour into skillet, lower heat to low, and simmer for 5 minutes, or until cooked through and slightly reduced. Add salt and pepper to taste.

Makes 4 servings

SERVING GUIDELINES

► **FOR GASTRIC SLEEVE AND BYPASS:**
  Week 1: Liquid diet.
  Weeks 2–4: Puree 2 ounces cooked meat with 2 tablespoons sauce.
  Weeks 5–7: Chop 2 ounces cooked meat and top with sauce.
  Weeks 8+: Serve 2–4 ounces cooked meat with sauce.

► **FOR BPD-DS:**
  Week 1: Liquid diet.
  Weeks 2–3: Puree 2 ounces cooked meat with 2 tablespoons sauce.
  Weeks 4+: Serve 3–4 ounces cooked meat with sauce.

► **FOR LAP-BAND:**
  Week 1: Liquid diet.
  Weeks 2–4: Puree 2 ounces cooked meat with 2 tablespoons sauce.
  Weeks 5–7: Chop 2 ounces cooked meat and top with sauce.
  Weeks 8+: Serve 2–4 ounces cooked meat with sauce.

► **FOR OTHERS:**
  Serve 4 ounces cooked meat with sauce.

Calories: 194, **Protein:** 25 g, **Fat:** 8 g, **Carbohydrates:** 5 g, **Cholesterol:** 76 mg, **Fiber:** 0 g, **Sodium:** 191 mg

Turkish Lamb and Cherry Tomatoes

If you like, you can make this recipe on skewers and you'll have shish kebab. By marinating the lamb in the spiced yogurt, it becomes incredibly tender.

¾ cup plain, fat-free yogurt
2 garlic cloves, finely minced
1 tablespoon tomato paste
½ teaspoon paprika
¼ teaspoon ground allspice
¼ teaspoon cinnamon
¼ teaspoon ground cumin
1 teaspoon dried thyme
¼ teaspoon cayenne pepper
1 pound lean lamb (tenderloin), cut into
  1-inch cubes
24 cherry tomatoes
Olive oil cooking spray
¾ cup low-sodium chicken broth

1. In a large bowl, stir together yogurt, garlic, tomato paste, and spices. Reserve 2 tablespoons to make sauce.
2. Add lamb, stirring to coat. Cover and marinate in refrigerator for 2 hours, stirring occasionally.
3. Preheat broiler and arrange rack to top position.
4. Spread lamb on broiling pan. Arrange tomatoes around lamb and spray with cooking spray.
5. Broil lamb for about 2 minutes, then turn and broil another 2 minutes. Tomatoes should be wilted.
6. While lamb and tomatoes are cooking, combine reserved marinade with chicken broth and simmer in a small saucepan for 3 minutes.
7. Pour over finished lamb and serve.

Makes 4 servings

SERVING GUIDELINES

► **FOR GASTRIC SLEEVE AND BYPASS:**
  Week 1: Liquid diet.
  Weeks 2–4: Puree 2 ounces cooked lamb and 4 tomatoes in 2 tablespoons sauce until smooth.
  Weeks 5–7: Chop 2 ounces cooked lamb and 4 tomatoes and top with sauce.
  Weeks 8+: Serve 2–4 ounces cooked lamb cubes and 4 tomatoes topped with sauce.

► **FOR BPD-DS:**
  Week 1: Liquid diet.
  Weeks 2–3: Puree 2 ounces cooked lamb and 4 tomatoes in 2 tablespoons sauce until smooth.
  Weeks 4+: Serve 3–4 ounces cooked lamb cubes and 4 tomatoes topped with sauce.

► **FOR LAP-BAND:**
  Week 1: Liquid diet.
  Weeks 2–4: Puree 2 ounces cooked lamb and 4 tomatoes in 2 tablespoons sauce until smooth.
  Weeks 5–7: Chop 2 ounces cooked lamb and 4 tomatoes and top with sauce.
  Weeks 8+: Serve 2–4 ounces cooked lamb cubes and 4 tomatoes topped with sauce.

► **FOR OTHERS:**
  Serve 4 ounces cooked lamb cubes and 6 tomatoes topped with sauce.

Calories: 235, **Protein:** 30 g, **Fat:** 8 g, **Carbohydrates:** 12 g, **Cholesterol:** 88 mg, **Fiber:** 2 g, **Sodium:** 162 mg

Grilled Salmon with Basil Seafood Sauce

I love salmon. It's one of those wonderful fish that can stand up to any spice or any sauce. This recipe pairs salmon with a sauce that smoothly combines very distinctive ingredients into one strong yet mellow flavor. The sauce can be refrigerated. If you're left with any extra sauce, try mixing it into canned tuna instead of plain mayo for lunch.

Olive oil cooking spray
1 pound salmon fillets
1 tablespoon light soy sauce

**Basil Seafood Sauce
(makes approximately 1 cup):**

½ cup fat-free sour cream
½ cup low-fat mayonnaise
2 tablespoons prepared horseradish
¼ cup chopped fresh basil
2 teaspoons light soy sauce
2 tablespoons minced dried onion
1 teaspoon minced fresh ginger
1 tablespoon anchovy paste

1. Preheat broiler and arrange rack to top position. Spray a broiling pan with cooking spray; place salmon on pan, skin side down, and coat with cooking spray.
2. Sprinkle salmon with soy sauce and broil for 5 to 7 minutes, or until cooked through but still moist.
3. *While salmon is broiling, make sauce:* Combine all sauce ingredients in a small bowl and mix well.
4. Either pour sauce over finished salmon or use it for dipping.

Makes 4 servings

SERVING GUIDELINES

- **FOR GASTRIC SLEEVE AND BYPASS:**
  Week 1: Liquid diet.
  Weeks 2–4: Puree 2 ounces cooked salmon fillet with 2 tablespoons sauce until smooth.
  Weeks 5+: Serve 2–4 ounces cooked salmon fillet topped with 2 tablespoons sauce.

- **FOR BPD-DS:**
  Week 1: Liquid diet.
  Weeks 2–3: Puree 2 ounces cooked salmon fillet with 2 tablespoons sauce until smooth.
  Weeks 4+: Serve 3–4 ounces cooked salmon fillet topped with 2 tablespoons sauce.

- **FOR LAP-BAND:**
  Week 1: Liquid diet.
  Weeks 2–4: Puree 2 ounces cooked salmon fillet with 2 tablespoons sauce until smooth.
  Weeks 5+: Serve 2–4 ounces cooked salmon fillet topped with 2 tablespoons sauce.

- **FOR OTHERS:**
  Serve 4 ounces cooked salmon fillet topped with 2 tablespoons sauce.

Salmon:

Calories: 193, **Protein:** 24 g, **Fat:** 10 g, **Carbohydrates:** 0 g, **Cholesterol:** 70 mg, **Fiber:** 0 g, **Sodium:** 197 mg

Basil Seafood Sauce (2 tablespoons):

Calories: 39, **Protein:** 1 g, **Fat:** 3 g, **Carbohydrates:** 3 g, **Cholesterol:** 7 mg, **Fiber:** 0 g, **Sodium:** 166 mg

Indian Spiced Salmon

The Indian style of cooking gives an authentic toasted spice flavor to this unusual salmon dish.

Spice mixture:

1 teaspoon ground coriander
1 teaspoon ground cumin
½ teaspoon ground turmeric
½ teaspoon dried thyme
½ teaspoon ground fennel seeds
¼ teaspoon ground black pepper
¼ teaspoon ground cinnamon
1 teaspoon ground cloves

1 pound salmon fillets
Butter-flavored cooking spray
⅓ cup plain, fat-free yogurt

1. *To make spice mixture:* Mix together spices on a flat plate.
2. Dredge fillets on both sides with spice mixture, patting gently to make it stick.
3. In a large nonstick skillet, heat cooking spray over medium-high heat just until it gets hot. Add fillets and cook for about 3 minutes on each side, or until medium rare. Remove fillets from pan and keep warm.
4. Add yogurt to hot pan and turn off heat. Stir to scrape up spice flavors left in pan.

Makes 4 servings

SERVING GUIDELINES

▶ **FOR GASTRIC SLEEVE AND BYPASS:**
Week 1: Liquid diet.
Weeks 2–4: Puree 2 ounces cooked salmon fillet with 2 tablespoons sauce until smooth.
Weeks 5+: Serve 2–4 ounces cooked salmon fillet topped with 2 tablespoons sauce.

▶ **FOR BPD-DS:**
Week 1: Liquid diet.
Weeks 2–3: Puree 2 ounces cooked salmon fillet with 2 tablespoons sauce until smooth.
Weeks 4+: Serve 3–4 ounces cooked salmon fillet topped with 2 tablespoons sauce.

▶ **FOR LAP-BAND:**
Week 1: Liquid diet.
Weeks 2–4: Puree 2 ounces cooked salmon fillet with 2 tablespoons sauce until smooth.
Weeks 5+: Serve 2–4 ounces cooked salmon fillet topped with 2 tablespoons sauce.

▶ **FOR OTHERS:**
Serve 4 ounces cooked salmon fillet topped with 2 tablespoons sauce.

Calories: 220, **Protein:** 26 g, **Fat:** 10 g, **Carbohydrates:** 4 g, **Cholesterol:** 71 mg, **Fiber:** 1 g, **Sodium:** 81 mg

Salmon with Wasabi Glaze and
Creamy Wasabi Sauce

Did you know that wasabi, often called Japanese mustard, is really a horseradish? Whatever you call it, it's fantastic with salmon.

Wasabi Glaze:

1 teaspoon wasabi paste
2 teaspoons light soy sauce
2 packets artificial sweetener
   (Splenda or Truvia)
1 tablespoon fresh lemon juice
1 large garlic clove, minced

Canola cooking spray
1 pound salmon fillet
Creamy Wasabi Sauce
(makes about 1/2 cup):

¼ cup fat-free sour cream
¼ cup low-fat mayonnaise
1½ teaspoons light soy sauce
½ packet artificial sweetener
1 teaspoon wasabi paste

1. *To make glaze:* In a small bowl, whisk all glaze ingredients together.
2. Preheat broiler and arrange rack to top position. Spray a broiling pan with cooking spray and place salmon in pan, skin side down.
3. Spread wasabi glaze on salmon fillet.
4. Broil for 7 to 10 minutes, depending on thickness of fish. To test for doneness, flake gently with a fork. It should be medium rare in middle.
5. *While salmon is broiling, make wasabi sauce:* Mix all sauce ingredients together until well blended. Either pour sauce over finished salmon or use it for dipping.

Makes 4 servings

SERVING GUIDELINES

- **FOR GASTRIC SLEEVE AND BYPASS:**
  Week 1: Liquid diet.
  Weeks 2–4: Puree 2 ounces cooked salmon fillet with 2 tablespoons sauce until smooth.
  Weeks 5+: Serve 2–4 ounces cooked salmon fillet topped with 2 tablespoons sauce.

- **FOR BPD-DS:**
  Week 1: Liquid diet.
  Weeks 2–3: Puree 2 ounces cooked salmon fillet with 2 tablespoons sauce until smooth.
  Weeks 4+: Serve 3–4 ounces cooked salmon fillet topped with 2 tablespoons sauce.

- **FOR LAP-BAND:**
  Week 1: Liquid diet.
  Weeks 2–4: Puree 2 ounces cooked salmon fillet with 2 tablespoons sauce until smooth.
  Weeks 5+: Serve 2–4 ounces cooked salmon fillet topped with 2 tablespoons sauce.

- **FOR OTHERS:**
  Serve 4 ounces cooked salmon fillet topped with 2 tablespoons sauce.

Salmon:

Calories: 199, **Protein:** 25 g, **Fat:** 10 g, **Carbohydrates:** 2 g, **Cholesterol:** 70 mg, **Fiber:** 0 g, **Sodium:** 169 mg

Wasabi Sauce (2 tablespoons):

Calories: 37, **Protein:** 1 g, **Fat:** 3 g, **Carbohydrates:** 3 g, **Cholesterol:** 4 mg, **Fiber:** 0 g, **Sodium:** 110 mg

Salmon with Creamy Lime-Dill Sauce

Salmon and dill are one of those natural combinations that's so good, it's never a cliché. Of course, we added a dollop of mustard to the sauce to make it unique.

Butter-flavored cooking spray
1 pound salmon fillet
¼ cup Dijon mustard
2 tablespoons fresh dill, or 1 tablespoon dried
2 tablespoons fat-free cream cheese
¼ cup fresh lime juice
½ teaspoon garlic powder
½ packet artificial sweetener (Splenda or Truvia)

1. Preheat broiler and arrange rack to top position. Spray broiler pan with cooking spray. Place salmon in pan, skin side down.
2. In a small bowl, combine half of mustard with half of dill and spread on salmon.
3. Broil salmon for 7 to 10 minutes, or until just medium rare in middle.
4. In another small bowl, combine remaining mustard and dill and remaining other sauce ingredients until creamy; pour over broiled fish to serve.

Makes 4 servings

SERVING GUIDELINES

► **FOR GASTRIC SLEEVE AND BYPASS:**
Week 1: Liquid diet.
Weeks 2–4: Puree 2 ounces cooked salmon fillet with 2 tablespoons sauce until smooth.
Weeks 5+: Serve 2–4 ounces cooked salmon fillet topped with 2 tablespoons sauce.

► **FOR BPD-DS:**
Week 1: Liquid diet.
Weeks 2–3: Puree 2 ounces cooked salmon fillet with 2 tablespoons sauce until smooth.
Weeks 4+: Serve 3–4 ounces cooked salmon fillet topped with 2 tablespoons sauce.

► **FOR LAP-BAND:**
Week 1: Liquid diet.
Weeks 2–4: Puree 2 ounces cooked salmon fillet with 2 tablespoons sauce until smooth.
Weeks 5+: Serve 2–4 ounces cooked salmon fillet topped with 2 tablespoons sauce.

► **FOR OTHERS:**
Serve 4 ounces cooked salmon fillet topped with 2 tablespoons sauce.

Calories: 231, **Protein:** 27 g, **Fat:** 11 g, **Carbohydrates:** 5 g, **Cholesterol:** 72 mg, **Fiber:** 2 g, **Sodium:** 174 mg

Salmon Croquettes with Spicy Tartar Sauce

These croquettes are kind of like tuna burgers, but a little more sophisticated.

1 (14-ounce) can pink salmon, drained
¼ cup gluten-free unseasoned panko crispy (Japanese-style bread crumbs)
½ cup egg substitute or 1 large egg, lightly beaten
2 tablespoons low-fat mayonnaise
1 tablespoon dried minced parsley
2 tablespoons dried minced onion
1 tablespoon dried celery leaves
1 teaspoon Worcestershire sauce
Olive oil cooking spray

Spicy Tartar Sauce:

½ cup low-fat mayonnaise
1 tablespoon sweet pickle relish
1 teaspoon fresh lemon juice
1 teaspoon prepared horseradish
½ teaspoon lemon-pepper

1. In a medium bowl, combine salmon with panko, egg substitute or egg, mayonnaise, parsley, onion, celery leaves, and Worcestershire. Mix until well blended, then divide and form into eight oval patties (croquettes).
2. Coat a large nonstick lidded skillet with cooking spray; heat over medium heat until hot but not smoking. Sauté patties for 3 to 4 minutes on one side until golden brown, flip, and sauté the other side until golden.
3. Cover skillet, lower heat to low, and cook for 7 minutes.
4. *While croquettes are cooking, make sauce:* In a small bowl, mix all sauce ingredients until combined well. Using a whisk, beat until light and creamy.

Makes 4 servings

SERVING GUIDELINES

► **FOR GASTRIC SLEEVE AND BYPASS:**
  Week 1: Liquid diet.
  Weeks 2–3: Puree 2 ounces croquettes with 2 tablespoons sauce.
  Weeks 4+: Serve 1–2 croquettes with 2 tablespoons sauce.

► **FOR BPD-DS:**
  Week 1: Liquid diet.
  Weeks 2–3: Puree 2 ounces croquettes with 2 tablespoons sauce.
  Weeks 4+: Serve 1–2 croquettes with 2 tablespoons sauce.

► **FOR LAP-BAND:**
  Week 1: Liquid diet.
  Weeks 2–3: Puree 2 ounces croquettes with 2 tablespoons sauce.
  Weeks 4+: Serve 1–2 croquettes with 2 tablespoons sauce.

► **FOR OTHERS:**
  Serve 2 croquettes with sauce.

Calories: 186, **Protein:** 24 g, **Fat:** 5 g, **Carbohydrates:** 14 g, **Cholesterol:** 99 mg, **Fiber:** 0 g, **Sodium:** 463 mg

Mustard-Crusted Halibut

Using ground soy nuts as a coating gives this classic recipe a luscious nutty flavor.

1 tablespoon Dijon mustard
1 tablespoon whole-grain mustard
1 teaspoon grated fresh lemon zest
1 teaspoon chopped fresh thyme, or ½
 teaspoons dried
1 tablespoon light soy sauce
1 pound halibut fillets, skinned
½ cup ground soy nuts
1 tablespoon chopped fresh parsley
Olive oil cooking spray
1 garlic clove, minced
1 cup bottled clam juice
Salt and pepper to taste

1. In a shallow bowl, combine mustards, lemon zest, thyme, and soy sauce. Dip fish and turn to coat both sides, then remove fish. Reserve mustard mixture.

2. On a flat plate, mix ground soy nuts and parsley and dredge coated fillets in mixture, turning to coat both sides.

3. Coat a medium nonstick skillet with cooking spray and sauté fish over medium heat for 2 minutes on each side. Lower heat to low and cook fish for 3 more minutes, or until just cooked through. Remove fish from pan and keep warm.

4. Sauté garlic in pan for 1 minute, or until golden. Stir clam juice and reserved mustard mixture into pan, scraping up any browned bits, and simmer for 3 minutes until slightly reduced. Add salt and pepper to taste.

Makes 4 servings

SERVING GUIDELINES

➤ **FOR GASTRIC SLEEVE AND BYPASS:**
 Week 1: Liquid diet.
 Weeks 2–4: Puree 2 ounces cooked fish with 2 tablespoons sauce until smooth.
 Weeks 5+: Serve 2–4 ounces cooked fish topped with 2 tablespoons sauce.

➤ **FOR BPD-DS:**
 Week 1: Liquid diet.
 Weeks 2–3: Puree 2 ounces cooked fish with 2 tablespoons sauce until smooth.
 Weeks 4+: Serve 3–4 ounces cooked fish topped with 2 tablespoons sauce.

➤ **FOR LAP-BAND:**
 Week 1: Liquid diet.
 Weeks 2–4: Puree 2 ounces cooked fish with 2 tablespoons sauce until smooth.
 Weeks 5+: Serve 2–4 ounces cooked fish topped with 2 tablespoons sauce.

➤ **FOR OTHERS:**
 Serve 4 ounces cooked fish topped with 2 tablespoons sauce.

Calories: 248, **Protein:** 33 g, **Fat:** 9 g, **Carbohydrates:** 9 g, **Cholesterol:** 36 mg, **Fiber:** 4 g, **Sodium:** 302 mg

Halibut with Piquant Tomato Sauce

The mild flavor of halibut seems to cry out for a really zesty sauce. This one gets an extra kick from curry paste.

Olive oil cooking spray
2 garlic cloves, minced
½ pound fresh mushrooms, thinly sliced
1¾ cups bottled clam juice
2 teaspoons red curry paste
¾ pound plum tomatoes, chopped
¼ cup chopped fresh basil
1 pound halibut fillet, skinned
Salt and pepper to taste

1. Coat medium nonstick lidded skillet with cooking spray and sauté garlic over medium heat for 1 minute, or until tender.
2. Add mushrooms, cover, and cook for 2 minutes, until just softened.
3. Stir in clam juice and curry paste. Add tomatoes and basil, lower heat, and simmer, covered, for 3 minutes, until tomatoes soften.
4. Add halibut, cover, and cook for 5 minutes, or until fish flakes easily with a fork. Add salt and pepper to taste.

Makes 4 servings

SERVING GUIDELINES

▶ **FOR GASTRIC SLEEVE AND BYPASS:**
   Week 1: Liquid diet.
   Weeks 2–4: Puree 2 ounces cooked fish with 2 tablespoons sauce until smooth.
   Weeks 5+: Serve 2–4 ounces cooked fish topped with 2 tablespoons sauce.

▶ **FOR BPD-DS:**
   Week 1: Liquid diet.
   Weeks 2–3: Puree 2 ounces cooked fish with 2 tablespoons sauce until smooth.
   Weeks 4+: Serve 3–4 ounces cooked fish topped with 2 tablespoons sauce.

▶ **FOR LAP-BAND:**
   Week 1: Liquid diet.
   Weeks 2–4: Puree 2 ounces cooked fish with 2 tablespoons sauce until smooth.
   Weeks 5+: Serve 2–4 ounces cooked fish topped with 2 tablespoons sauce.

▶ **FOR OTHERS:**
   Serve 4 ounces cooked fish topped with 2 tablespoons sauce.

Calories: 169, **Protein:** 27 g, **Fat:** 3 g, **Carbohydrates:** 7 g, **Cholesterol:** 36 mg, **Fiber:** 2 g, **Sodium:** 260 mg

Souvlaki-Style Swordfish

Even though the Greeks cook a lot of fish, we've never seen it served with a traditional sou-vlaki sauce before. I don't know why; it seems to be such a perfect combination of flavors.

1 tablespoon fresh lemon juice
½ teaspoon dried oregano
½ teaspoon freshly ground black pepper
1 pound skinless swordfish steaks
1 large cucumber, peeled, seeded, and grated
1 cup plain, fat-free yogurt
1½ teaspoons chopped fresh mint leaves
½ teaspoon chopped garlic
Olive oil cooking spray

1. Combine lemon juice, oregano, and pepper and sprinkle over fish. Cover and marinate in refrigerator for 15 minutes.
2. Wrap grated cucumber in a double layer of paper towels and squeeze to extract liquid.
3. Put cucumber, yogurt, mint, and garlic in a food processor and puree until smooth.
4. Preheat broiler and place rack in top position. Coat a nonstick broiler pan with cooking spray. Place fish on pan and broil, turning once, for about 4 minutes on each side, or until just cooked through.

Makes 4 servings

SERVING GUIDELINES

► **FOR GASTRIC SLEEVE AND BYPASS:**
   Week 1: Liquid diet.
   Weeks 2–4: Puree 2 ounces cooked fish with 2 tablespoons sauce until smooth.
   Weeks 5+: Serve 2–4 ounces cooked fish topped with 2 tablespoons sauce.

► **FOR BPD-DS:**
   Week 1: Liquid diet.
   Weeks 2–3: Puree 2 ounces cooked fish with 2 tablespoons sauce until smooth.
   Weeks 4+: Serve 3–4 ounces cooked fish topped with 2 tablespoons sauce.

► **FOR LAP-BAND:**
   Week 1: Liquid diet.
   Weeks 2–4: Puree 2 ounces cooked fish with 2 tablespoons sauce until smooth.
   Weeks 5+: Serve 2–4 ounces cooked fish topped with 2 tablespoons sauce.

► **FOR OTHERS:**
   Serve 4 ounces cooked fish topped with 2 tablespoons sauce.

Calories: 204, **Protein:** 27 g, **Fat:** 5 g, **Carbohydrates:** 12 g, **Cholesterol:** 46 mg, **Fiber:** 1 g, **Sodium:** 185 mg

Tangy Swordfish and Tomatoes

The beauty of swordfish is that it's flavorful enough to stand up to the most assertive sauces, like this one spiked with mustard and tarragon.

Olive oil cooking spray
1 pound swordfish steak
1½ cups chopped fresh tomatoes
2 teaspoons light soy sauce
1 tablespoon Dijon mustard
2½ teaspoons chopped fresh tarragon, or
   ¾ teaspoon dried
Salt and pepper to taste

1. In a medium nonstick skillet, heat cooking spray over high heat until hot but not smoking; sear swordfish for 2 minutes on each side.
2. Lower heat to medium and pour tomatoes around fish. Drizzle fish with soy sauce, cover, and cook for 5 minutes. Remove fish from skillet and keep warm.
3. Add mustard and tarragon to tomatoes and stir well to combine. Add salt and pepper to taste.

Makes 4 servings

SERVING GUIDELINES

► **FOR GASTRIC SLEEVE AND BYPASS:**
  Week 1: Liquid diet.
  Weeks 2–4: Puree 2 ounces cooked fish with 2 tablespoons sauce until smooth.
  Weeks 5+: Serve 2–4 ounces cooked fish topped with 2 tablespoons sauce.

► **FOR BPD-DS:**
  Week 1: Liquid diet.
  Weeks 2–3: Puree 2 ounces cooked fish with 2 tablespoons sauce until smooth.
  Weeks 4+: Serve 3–4 ounces cooked fish topped with 2 tablespoons sauce.

► **FOR LAP-BAND:**
  Week 1: Liquid diet.
  Weeks 2–4: Puree 2 ounces cooked fish with 2 tablespoons sauce until smooth.
  Weeks 5+: Serve 2–4 ounces cooked fish topped with 2 tablespoons sauce.

► **FOR OTHERS:**
  Serve 4 ounces cooked fish topped with 2 tablespoons sauce.

Calories: 159, **Protein:** 23 g, **Fat:** 5 g, **Carbohydrates:** 4 g, **Cholesterol:** 45 mg, **Fiber:** 1 g, **Sodium:** 235 mg

Sole with White Wine and Capers

This simple yet elegant way of cooking sole also works with any delicate, white-fleshed fish, such as tilapia or flounder.

Olive oil cooking spray
¼ cup minced shallots
½ cup white wine
1 teaspoon capers, drained
1 pound skinless sole fillets
Salt and pepper to taste

1. Coat bottom of a medium nonstick skillet with cooking spray; heat over medium heat and sauté shallots until lightly browned.
2. Add wine and capers to pan and bring to simmer.
3. Place fish fillets in pan, cover, and poach for 3 minutes, or until fish flakes easily with a fork. Add salt and pepper to taste.

Makes 4 servings

SERVING GUIDELINES

► **FOR GASTRIC SLEEVE AND BYPASS:**
Week 1: Liquid diet.
Weeks 2–4: Puree 2 ounces cooked fish with 2 tablespoons sauce until smooth.
Weeks 5+: Serve 2–4 ounces cooked fish topped with 2 tablespoons sauce.

► **FOR BPD-DS:**
Week 1: Liquid diet.
Weeks 2–3: Puree 2 ounces cooked fish with 2 tablespoons sauce until smooth.
Weeks 4+: Serve 3–4 ounces cooked fish topped with 2 tablespoons sauce.

► **FOR LAP-BAND:**
Week 1: Liquid diet.
Weeks 2–4: Puree 2 ounces cooked fish with 2 tablespoons sauce until smooth.
Weeks 5+: Serve 2–4 ounces cooked fish topped with 2 tablespoons sauce.

► **FOR OTHERS:**
Serve 4 ounces cooked fish topped with 2 tablespoons sauce.

Calories: 131, **Protein:** 22 g, **Fat:** 1 g, **Carbohydrates:** 2 g, **Cholesterol:** 54 mg, **Fiber:** 0 g, **Sodium:** 121 mg

Bluefish with Mustard-Horseradish Glaze

You need a fish with an assertive flavor of its own to stand up to this pungent glaze. I think bluefish is perfect—but it also works with swordfish or salmon. We adapted this recipe from *The Legal Sea Foods Cookbook*.

1 pound bluefish fillets

Olive oil cooking spray

¼ cup light mayonnaise

1 tablespoon prepared horseradish

2 tablespoons Dijon mustard

¼ cup minced shallots

2 teaspoons Worcestershire sauce

2 tablespoons minced dried parsley, plus
more for serving

1. Preheat broiler and arrange rack to top position. Place fillets, skin side down, in broiling pan and coat lightly with cooking spray.
2. Broil bluefish for 6 minutes, or until almost done.
3. While fish is broiling, combine mayonnaise, horseradish, mustard, shallots, Worcestershire, and parsley in a small bowl.
4. Remove fish from broiler, spread lightly with sauce, and continue to broil for about 3 minutes, or until lightly browned. Sprinkle with parsley and serve.

Makes 4 servings

SERVING GUIDELINES

▶ **FOR GASTRIC SLEEVE AND BYPASS:**
Week 1: Liquid diet.
Weeks 2–4: Puree 2 ounces cooked fish with 2 tablespoons sauce until smooth.
Weeks 5+: Serve 2–4 ounces cooked fish topped with 2 tablespoons sauce.

▶ **FOR BPD-DS:**
Week 1: Liquid diet.
Weeks 2–3: Puree 2 ounces cooked fish with 2 tablespoons sauce until smooth.
Weeks 4+: Serve 3–4 ounces cooked fish topped with 2 tablespoons sauce.

▶ **FOR LAP-BAND:**
Week 1: Liquid diet.
Weeks 2–4: Puree 2 ounces cooked fish with 2 tablespoons sauce until smooth.
Weeks 5+: Serve 2–4 ounces cooked fish topped with 2 tablespoons sauce.

▶ **FOR OTHERS:**
Serve 4 ounces cooked fish topped with 2 tablespoons sauce.

Calories: 219, **Protein:** 25 g, **Fat:** 12 g, **Carbohydrates:** 6 g, **Cholesterol:** 72 mg, **Fiber:** 0 g, **Sodium:** 305 mg

Cajun-Spiced Catfish with Citrus-Horseradish Sauce

We love the spiciness of this fish, especially when it's contrasted with a tangy lemon-lime sauce.

1 pound skinless catfish fillets
2 teaspoons paprika
1 garlic clove, minced
1 teaspoon dried oregano
1 teaspoon dried thyme
½ teaspoon cayenne pepper
Olive oil cooking spray
    Citrus-Horseradish Sauce
    (makes a little over 1/2 cup):
¼ cup low-fat mayonnaise
¼ cup fat-free sour cream
½ teaspoon grated lemon zest
1½ teaspoons fresh lemon juice
½ teaspoon grated lime zest
1½ teaspoons fresh lime juice
1 teaspoon capers, drained
1 teaspoon prepared horseradish
¼ cup chopped fresh basil leaves

1. Place fish on flat plate. Combine paprika, garlic, oregano, thyme, and cayenne thoroughly and rub on fish. Cover with foil and refrigerate for 20 minutes.
2. *While fish is chilling, make sauce:* Combine all sauce ingredients in a medium bowl and whisk until smooth.
3. Preheat broiler and arrange rack to top position. Coat a nonstick broiling pan with cooking spray, place fish on it, and broil for 4 minutes, or until fish flakes easily with a fork. Serve with sauce.

Makes 4 servings

SERVING GUIDELINES

- **FOR GASTRIC SLEEVE AND BYPASS:**
  Week 1: Liquid diet.
  Weeks 2–4: Puree 2 ounces cooked fish with 2 tablespoons sauce until smooth.
  Weeks 5+: Serve 2–4 ounces cooked fish topped with 2 tablespoons sauce.

- **FOR BPD-DS:**
  Week 1: Liquid diet.
  Weeks 2–3: Puree 2 ounces cooked fish with 2 tablespoons sauce until smooth.
  Weeks 4+: Serve 3–4 ounces cooked fish topped with 2 tablespoons sauce.

- **FOR LAP-BAND:**
  Week 1: Liquid diet.
  Weeks 2–4: Puree 2 ounces cooked fish with 2 tablespoons sauce until smooth.
  Weeks 5+: Serve 2–4 ounces cooked fish topped with 2 tablespoons sauce.

- **FOR OTHERS:**
  Serve 4 ounces cooked fish topped with 2 tablespoons sauce.

Catfish:

Calories: 125, **Protein:** 21 g, **Fat:** 4 g, **Carbohydrates:** 1 g, **Cholesterol:** 66 mg, **Fiber:** 0 g, **Sodium:** 90 mg

Citrus-Horseradish Sauce (2 tablespoons):

Calories: 35, **Protein:** 1 g, **Fat:** 3 g, **Carbohydrates:** 2 g, **Cholesterol:** 4 mg, **Fiber:** 0 g, **Sodium:** 84 mg

Seared Tuna over Sesame Spinach

Want a quick, tasty recipe that works as well on a work night as it does for company? Try this dish, but make sure that you use a good, fresh tuna.

2 tablespoons low-sodium soy sauce
1 tablespoon fresh lime juice
½ teaspoon cayenne pepper
½ teaspoon salt
1 pound fresh tuna (about 1 inch thick)
1 (16-ounce) bag frozen chopped spinach
1 teaspoon sesame oil
1 tablespoon toasted sesame seeds
(optional)

1. In a bowl or resealable plastic bag large enough to hold fish, combine soy sauce, lime juice, cayenne, and salt.
2. Add tuna, making sure that it's completely coated. Close bag or tightly cover bowl and marinate in refrigerator for 15 to 30 minutes.
3. While tuna is marinating, prepare spinach in microwave according to package directions. Toss with sesame oil and sesame seeds (if using).
4. Remove tuna from marinade and let excess drip off.
5. Heat a medium skillet over a medium-high heat. Sear tuna for 2 to 3 minutes on each side for medium rare, then slice into ½-inch-thick slices. Serve over spinach.

Makes 4 servings

▶ **Cooking Tip**: To toast your own sesame seeds, toast in a toaster oven on the lightest toast setting for 30 seconds to 1 minute, or toast in a dry skillet over medium heat for 1 minute, or until light golden brown.

SERVING GUIDELINES

▶ **FOR GASTRIC SLEEVE AND BYPASS:**
  Week 1: Liquid diet.
  Weeks 2–3: Puree 2 ounces cooked tuna and spinach.
  Weeks 4+: Serve 2–4 ounces cooked tuna and spinach.

▶ **FOR BPD-DS:**
  Week 1: Liquid diet.
  Weeks 2–3: Puree 2 ounces cooked tuna and spinach.
  Weeks 4+: Serve 2–4 ounces cooked tuna and spinach.

▶ **FOR LAP-BAND:**
  Week 1: Liquid diet.
  Weeks 2–3: Puree 2 ounces cooked tuna and spinach.
  Weeks 4+: Serve 2–4 ounces cooked tuna and spinach.

▶ **FOR OTHERS:**
  Serve 4 ounces cooked tuna and spinach.

Calories: 259, **Protein:** 36 g, **Fat:** 9 g, **Carbohydrates:** 3 g, **Cholesterol:** 56 mg, **Fiber:** 0 g, **Sodium:** 350 mg

Tuna Mousse

If you think tuna salad is boring, wait until you taste this recipe. It's terrific for lunch or for a light summer supper.

2 (6-ounce) cans tuna packed in water, drained
2 tablespoons low-fat mayonnaise
2 tablespoons fat-free sour cream
2 tablespoons fat-free cream cheese, softened
½ cup diced shallots
1 tablespoon fresh lemon juice
¼ teaspoon ground pepper
½ teaspoon celery seeds
2 tablespoons chopped fresh parsley

1. In a food processor, combine all ingredients, except parsley, and pulse until smooth.
2. Add parsley and pulse just until combined.
3. Transfer mousse to a bowl and refrigerate for at least 1 hour before serving.

Makes 4 servings

SERVING GUIDELINES

► **FOR GASTRIC SLEEVE AND BYPASS:**
   Week 1: Liquid diet.
   Weeks 2+: Serve ¼–½ cup mousse as is.

► **FOR BPD-DS:**
   Week: 1: Liquid diet.
   Weeks 2+: Serve ¼–½ cup mousse as is.

► **FOR LAP-BAND:**
   Week 1: Liquid diet.
   Weeks 2+: Serve ¼–½ cup mousse as is.

► **FOR OTHERS:**
   Serve ½ cup mousse as is.

Calories: 154, **Protein:** 23 g, **Fat:** 4 g, **Carbohydrates:** 9 g, **Cholesterol:** 5 mg, **Fiber:** 0 g, **Sodium:** 486 mg

Quick Fish Mock Tacos with Jalapeño Lime Crema

Here's my low-carb twist on yummy fish taco—try wrapping the fish and toppings in crisp lettuce leaves.

Canola cooking spray
Jalapeño Lime Crema:
¼ cup chopped scallions or green onions
1 fresh jalapeño pepper, seeded and minced
½ cup cilantro, half shredded, half saved as whole leaves for serving
¼ cup fat-free mayonnaise
¼ cup fat-free sour cream
1 teaspoon grated fresh lime zest
1½ teaspoons fresh lime juice
¼ teaspoon salt
1 garlic clove, minced

1 teaspoon ground cumin
1 teaspoon ground coriander
1 teaspoon smoked paprika
½ teaspoon cayenne pepper
1 pound firm white fish fillets, such as red snapper or tilapia
Iceberg lettuce leaves
1 medium avocado, peeled, pitted, and sliced thinly
½ cup salsa verde

1. Preheat oven to 425°F and spray a baking sheet with cooking spray.
2. *To make crema:* Thoroughly combine all crema ingredients in a small bowl; set aside.
3. Combine cumin, coriander, paprika, and cayenne and rub onto fish fillets.
4. Place fish on prepared baking sheet and bake for 9 to 12 minutes, or until fish flakes easily with a fork. Remove from oven and flake fish into smaller pieces.
5. In each lettuce leaf, place ½ cup of fish, 1 to 2 slices of avocado, and reserved cilantro leaves.
6. Top with 1 tablespoon of crema and 2 tablespoons salsa verde.

Makes 4–6 servings

SERVING GUIDELINES

▸ **FOR GASTRIC SLEEVE AND BYPASS:**
Week 1: Liquid diet.
Weeks 2–3: Puree 2 ounces cooked fish with 2
tablespoons avocado, crema, and salsa.
Weeks 4–7: Chop 2 ounces cooked fish and top
with 2 tablespoons avocado, crema, and salsa.
Weeks 8+: Serve 2–4 ounces cooked fish in
lettuce wrap, topped with 2 tablespoons
avocado, crema, and salsa.

▸ **FOR BPD-DS:**
Week 1: Liquid diet.
Weeks 2–3: Puree 2 ounces cooked fish with 2
tablespoons avocado, crema, and salsa.
Weeks 4–7: Chop 2 ounces cooked fish and top
with 2 tablespoons avocado, crema, and salsa.
Weeks 8+: Serve 2–4 ounces cooked fish in
lettuce wrap, topped with 2 tablespoons
avocado, crema, and salsa.

▸ **FOR LAP-BAND:**
Week 1: Liquid diet.
Weeks 2–3: Puree 2 ounces cooked fish with 2
tablespoons avocado, crema, and salsa.
Weeks 4–7: Chop 2 ounces cooked fish and top
with 2 tablespoons avocado, crema, and salsa.
Weeks 8+: Serve 2–4 ounces cooked fish in
lettuce wrap, topped with 2 tablespoons
avocado, crema, and salsa.

▸ **FOR OTHERS:**
Serve 4 ounces cooked fish in lettuce wrap,
topped with avocado, crema, and salsa.

Calories: 258, **Protein:** 32 g, **Fat:** 8 g, **Carbohydrates:** 11 g, **Cholesterol:** 64 mg, **Fiber:** 5 g, **Sodium:** 515 mg

Balinese Shrimp

Exotically spiced, sweet, and tangy, this creamy seafood recipe layers lots of sophisticated flavors, but it's simple enough to prepare for a weeknight dinner.

Canola cooking spray

8 garlic cloves, minced

¾ cup water

1 teaspoon ground cumin

1 teaspoon ground coriander

½ teaspoon ground turmeric

1 pound large shrimp, peeled and deveined

1 cup plain, fat-free yogurt

2 tablespoons dried chives

2 packets artificial sweetener (Splenda or Truvia)

1. In a large nonstick lidded skillet, heat cooking spray over medium heat until hot but not smoking. Add garlic and sauté until golden, about 30 seconds.
2. Stir in water, cumin, coriander, and turmeric; cover, lower heat, and simmer for 7 minutes.
3. Add shrimp and cook, uncovered, stirring, for 3 minutes, or until they turn pink.
4. Stir in yogurt, chives, and sweetener and simmer over very low heat for 2 minutes, stirring occasionally.

Makes 4 servings

SERVING GUIDELINES

► **FOR GASTRIC SLEEVE AND BYPASS:**
Week 1: Liquid diet.
Weeks 2–4: Puree 2 ounces cooked shrimp with 2 tablespoons sauce.
Weeks 5–7: Chop 2 ounces cooked shrimp and top with sauce.
Weeks 8+: Serve 2–4 ounces cooked shrimp with sauce.

► **FOR BPD-DS:**
Week 1: Liquid diet.
Weeks 2–3: Puree 2 ounces cooked shrimp with 2 tablespoons sauce.
Weeks 4+: Serve 3–4 ounces cooked shrimp topped with sauce.

► **FOR LAP-BAND:**
Week 1: Liquid diet.
Weeks 2–4: Puree 2 ounces cooked shrimp with 2 tablespoons sauce.
Weeks 5–7: Chop 2 ounces cooked shrimp and top with sauce.
Weeks 8+: Serve 2–4 ounces cooked shrimp with sauce.

► **FOR OTHERS:**
Serve 4 ounces cooked shrimp topped with sauce.

Calories: 180, **Protein:** 28 g, **Fat:** 2 g, **Carbohydrates:** 11 g, **Cholesterol:** 174 mg, **Fiber:** 1 g, **Sodium:** 234 mg

Chilled Shrimp with Ponzu Sauce

Ponzu, the traditional Japanese sauce, gives this light summery dish a sweetly spicy kick.

1 pound large shrimp, peeled and
   deveined

Ponzu Sauce:

2 tablespoons light soy sauce
2 tablespoons fresh orange juice
2 tablespoons fresh lime juice
Brown-sugar artificial sweetener
   (2 teaspoons equivalent)
½ teaspoon Asian chili paste with garlic
1 tablespoon minced fresh ginger
¼ cup chopped fresh basil

1. In a large pot, bring 4 quarts of water to a rapid boil, add shrimp, and cook for 1 minute.
2. Drain shrimp and immediately transfer to a bowl of ice water. When chilled, drain shrimp and refrigerate.
3. *To make sauce:* In a small bowl, combine all sauce ingredients. (Sauce can be refrigerated until ready to use, up to 10 hours.) Toss shrimp with sauce 10 minutes before serving.

Makes 4 servings

SERVING GUIDELINES

▶ **FOR GASTRIC SLEEVE AND BYPASS:**
   Week 1: Liquid diet.
   Weeks 2–4: Puree 2 ounces cooked shrimp with 2 tablespoons sauce.
   Weeks 5–7: Chop 2 ounces cooked shrimp and top with sauce.
   Weeks 8+: Serve 2–4 ounces cooked shrimp with sauce.

▶ **FOR BPD-DS:**
   Week 1: Liquid diet.
   Weeks 2–3: Puree 2 ounces cooked shrimp with 2 tablespoons sauce.
   Weeks 4+: Serve 3–4 ounces cooked shrimp topped with sauce.

▶ **FOR LAP-BAND:**
   Week 1: Liquid diet.
   Weeks 2–4: Puree 2 ounces cooked shrimp with 2 tablespoons sauce.
   Weeks 5–7: Chop 2 ounces cooked shrimp and top with sauce.
   Weeks 8+: Serve 2–4 ounces cooked shrimp with sauce.

▶ **FOR OTHERS:**
   Serve 4 ounces cooked shrimp topped with sauce.

Calories: 140, **Protein:** 24 g, **Fat:** 2 g, **Carbohydrates:** 4 g, **Cholesterol:** 173 mg, **Fiber:** 0 g, **Sodium:** 448 mg

Shrimp in Green Sauce

This is a classic Spanish shrimp recipe that uses lots of garlic, fresh herbs, and a little heat, without all the fat of the original.

4 garlic cloves, peeled
1 teaspoon olive oil
4 scallions, trimmed and chopped
¾ cup fresh parsley (leaves and thin stems)
1 pound shrimp, peeled and deveined
½ teaspoon crushed red pepper flakes, or to taste
½ cup bottled clam juice
¼ cup water
2 teaspoons cornstarch

1. Combine garlic and olive oil in a small food processor and blend until it forms a paste. Add scallions and parsley and pulse until minced.
2. Toss garlic-herb mixture with shrimp and red pepper flakes.
3. Put shrimp into a large skillet and add clam juice. Cook over high heat, stirring once, until shrimp is cooked, 5 to 7 minutes. Remove shrimp from skillet and keep warm.
4. In a small bowl, combine water with cornstarch and whisk until smooth. Stir cornstarch mixture into garlic and herb mixture in skillet, lower heat to low, and simmer, stirring, until sauce thickens, 5 to 7 minutes.
5. Add shrimp into sauce, turning to coat.

Makes 4 servings

SERVING GUIDELINES

► **FOR GASTRIC SLEEVE AND BYPASS:**
Week 1: Liquid diet.
Weeks 2–3: Puree 2 ounces cooked shrimp with 2 tablespoons sauce.
Weeks 4–7: Chop 2 ounces cooked shrimp and top with 2 tablespoons sauce.
Weeks 8+: Serve 2–4 ounces cooked shrimp with 2 tablespoons sauce.

► **FOR BPD-DS:**
Week 1: Liquid diet.
Weeks 2–3: Puree 2 ounces cooked shrimp with 2 tablespoons sauce.
Weeks 4–7: Chop 2 ounces cooked shrimp and top with 2 tablespoons sauce.
Weeks 8+: Serve 2–4 ounces cooked shrimp with 2 tablespoons sauce.

► **FOR LAP-BAND:**
Week 1: Liquid diet.
Weeks 2–3: Puree 2 ounces cooked shrimp with 2 tablespoons sauce.
Weeks 4–7: Chop 2 ounces cooked shrimp and top with 2 tablespoons sauce.
Weeks 8+: Serve 2–4 ounces cooked shrimp with 2 tablespoons sauce.

► **FOR OTHERS:**
Serve 4 ounces cooked shrimp with sauce.

Calories: 121, **Protein:** 24 g, **Fat:** 2 g, **Carbohydrates:** 3 g, **Cholesterol:** 183 mg, **Fiber:** 1 g, **Sodium:** 234 mg

Shrimp Calypso

Tangy with a creamy yogurt and pineapple sauce, this recipe gets its tropical heat from typical island spicing. This dish can be served hot or cold.

1 pound large shrimp, peeled and deveined
1 teaspoon crushed red pepper flakes
1 teaspoon ground turmeric
1 teaspoon grated fresh ginger
2 garlic cloves, minced
1 cup plain, fat-free yogurt
½ cup chopped green onions or scallions
Canola cooking spray
½ cup diced fresh pineapple
1 tablespoon chopped fresh cilantro

1. Combine shrimp, crushed red pepper, turmeric, ginger, garlic, yogurt, and green onions in a large resealable plastic bag. Seal and turn to coat all shrimp, then marinate in refrigerator for 30 minutes.
2. Coat bottom of a large skillet with cooking spray and heat over medium heat until hot. Pour shrimp and marinade into skillet and cook, stirring, for 3 minutes, or until shrimp turn pink.
3. Stir in pineapple and cook for 2 minutes. Sprinkle with cilantro and serve.

Makes 4 servings

SERVING GUIDELINES

► **FOR GASTRIC SLEEVE AND BYPASS:**
Week 1: Liquid diet.
Weeks 2–4: Puree 2 ounces cooked shrimp with 2 tablespoons sauce.
Weeks 5–7: Chop 2 ounces cooked shrimp and top with sauce.
Weeks 8+: Serve 2–4 ounces cooked shrimp with sauce.

► **FOR BPD-DS:**
Week 1: Liquid diet.
Weeks 2–3: Puree 2 ounces cooked shrimp with 2 tablespoons sauce.
Weeks 4+: Serve 3–4 ounces cooked shrimp topped with sauce.

► **FOR LAP-BAND:**
Week 1: Liquid diet.
Weeks 2–4: Puree 2 ounces cooked shrimp with 2 tablespoons sauce.
Weeks 5–7: Chop 2 ounces cooked shrimp and top with sauce.
Weeks 8+: Serve 2–4 ounces cooked shrimp with sauce.

► **FOR OTHERS:**
Serve 4 ounces cooked shrimp topped with sauce.

Calories: 184, **Protein:** 28 g, **Fat:** 2 g, **Carbohydrates:** 12 g, **Cholesterol:** 174 mg, **Fiber:** 1 g, **Sodium:** 234 mg

Shrimp Italiano

This recipe is based on one that I have been making for years—Italian vegetable stew. It's sort of like a French ratatouille without the eggplant. It can be served hot or cold.

Olive oil cooking spray

¾ cup coarsely chopped onion

3 large garlic cloves, minced

½ pound fresh white mushrooms, cut into eighths

1 small zucchini, cut coarsely into cubes (about 1 cup)

1 cup coarsely chopped and seeded bell pepper

1 (14.5-ounce) can diced tomatoes

¼ cup dry red wine

1½ teaspoons minced fresh basil, or ¾ teaspoons dried

½ teaspoon red pepper flakes

1 pound large shrimp, peeled and deveined

Salt and pepper to taste

1. Coat bottom of a large pot with cooking spray and sauté onion, garlic, and mushrooms over medium heat for 5 to 7 minutes, or until just translucent.
2. Add all other ingredients, except shrimp, salt, and pepper. Cover pot and cook over low heat for 2 hours.
3. Add shrimp, cover pot, and simmer for 3 minutes, or until shrimp turn pink. Add salt and pepper to taste.

Makes 4 servings

SERVING GUIDELINES

► **FOR GASTRIC SLEEVE AND BYPASS:**
Week 1: Liquid diet.
Weeks 2–4: Puree 2 ounces cooked shrimp with ¼ cup vegetables.
Weeks 5–7: Chop 2 ounces cooked shrimp and serve with ¼ cup vegetables.
Weeks 8+: Serve 2–4 ounces shrimp with ¼ cup vegetables.

► **FOR BPD-DS:**
Week 1: Liquid diet.
Weeks 2–3: Puree 2 ounces cooked shrimp with ¼ cup vegetables.
Weeks 4+: Serve 3–4 ounces shrimp with ½ cup vegetables.

► **FOR LAP-BAND:**
Week 1: Liquid diet.
Weeks 2–4: Puree 2 ounces cooked shrimp with ¼ cup vegetables.
Weeks 5–7: Chop 2 ounces cooked shrimp and serve with ¼ cup vegetables.
Weeks 8+: Serve 2–4 ounces shrimp with ¼ cup vegetables.

► **FOR OTHERS:**
Serve 4 ounces shrimp with ½–1 cup vegetables.

Calories: 219, **Protein:** 28 g, **Fat:** 2 g, **Carbohydrates:** 17 g, **Cholesterol:** 172 mg, **Fiber:** 4 g, **Sodium:** 335 mg

Shrimp Scampi

If you think that scampi without lots of olive oil or butter isn't possible, try this recipe. It has all the flavor of a traditional scampi, but it's lighter and brighter.

Olive oil cooking spray
½ cup minced shallots
3 garlic cloves, minced
1 pound large shrimp, peeled and deveined
½ cup white wine
¼ cup bottled clam juice
¼ cup chopped fresh parsley
2 tablespoons fresh lemon juice
Salt and pepper to taste

1. In a large nonstick skillet, heat cooking spray over medium-high heat until hot but not smoking. Sauté shallots and garlic for 1 minute, or until barely golden.
2. Add shrimp and sauté until they just turn pink, 2 to 3 minutes. Remove shrimp from pan.
3. Stir in wine and clam juice and bring to a boil. Lower heat to medium and cook for 30 seconds.
4. Place shrimp back in pan, and add parsley and lemon juice. Toss well to coat shrimp and cook for 1 minute. Add salt and pepper to taste.

Makes 4 servings

SERVING GUIDELINES

► **FOR GASTRIC SLEEVE AND BYPASS:**
  Week 1: Liquid diet.
  Weeks 2–4: Puree 2 ounces cooked shrimp with 2 tablespoons sauce.
  Weeks 5–7: Chop 2 ounces cooked shrimp and top with sauce.
  Weeks 8+: Serve 2–4 ounces cooked shrimp with sauce.

► **FOR BPD-DS:**
  Week 1: Liquid diet.
  Weeks 2–3: Puree 2 ounces cooked shrimp with 2 tablespoons sauce.
  Weeks 4+: Serve 3–4 ounces cooked shrimp topped with sauce.

► **FOR LAP-BAND:**
  Week 1: Liquid diet.
  Weeks 2–4: Puree 2 ounces cooked shrimp with 2 tablespoons sauce.
  Weeks 5–7: Chop 2 ounces cooked shrimp and top with sauce.
  Weeks 8+: Serve 2–4 ounces cooked shrimp with sauce.

► **FOR OTHERS:**
  Serve 4 ounces cooked shrimp topped with sauce.

Calories: 162, **Protein:** 24 g, **Fat:** 2 g, **Carbohydrates:** 6 g, **Cholesterol:** 172 mg, **Fiber:** 0 g, **Sodium:** 193 mg

Shrimp with Coconut-Curry Tomato Sauce

Here's a creamy, spicy shrimp curry that's so full of authentic flavor, it's hard to believe that we're allowed to eat it.

Canola cooking spray

½ cup thinly sliced onion

3 garlic cloves, minced

1 small jalapeño pepper, seeded and chopped

1½ teaspoons minced fresh ginger

1½ teaspoons mild curry powder

1 (28-ounce) can diced tomatoes with their juice

1 (14-ounce) can light unsweetened coconut milk

1 packet artificial sweetener (Splenda or Truvia)

1 pound fresh large shrimp, peeled and deveined

1. In a large nonstick skillet, heat cooking spray over medium heat until hot but not smoking. Sauté onion, garlic, jalapeño, and ginger for about 5 minutes, or until soft. Add curry powder and cook until fragrant, about 30 seconds.

2. Add tomatoes with their juice, coconut milk, and sweetener. Lower heat and simmer over low heat for about 15 minutes, or until slightly thickened.

3. Add shrimp and cook, stirring, for 3 to 5 minutes, or until shrimps turn pink and opaque.

Makes 4 servings

SERVING GUIDELINES

➤ **FOR GASTRIC SLEEVE AND BYPASS:**
Week 1: Liquid diet.
Weeks 2–4: Puree 2 ounces cooked shrimp with 2 tablespoons sauce.
Weeks 5–7: Chop 2 ounces cooked shrimp and top with sauce.
Weeks 8+: Serve 2–4 ounces cooked shrimp with sauce.

➤ **FOR BPD-DS:**
Week 1: Liquid diet.
Weeks 2–3: Puree 2 ounces cooked shrimp with 2 tablespoons sauce.
Weeks 4+: Serve 3–4 ounces cooked shrimp topped with sauce.

➤ **FOR LAP-BAND:**
Week 1: Liquid diet.
Weeks 2–4: Puree 2 ounces cooked shrimp with 2 tablespoons sauce.
Weeks 5–7: Chop 2 ounces cooked shrimp and top with sauce.
Weeks 8+: Serve 2–4 ounces cooked shrimp with sauce.

➤ **FOR OTHERS:**
Serve 4 ounces cooked shrimp topped with sauce.

Calories: 284, **Protein:** 27 g, **Fat:** 9 g, **Carbohydrates:** 20 g, **Cholesterol:** 172 mg, **Fiber:** 4 g, **Sodium:** 504 mg

Singapore Shrimp Dumplings

Even though these delicate dumplings use cabbage leaves instead of traditional dough wrappers, they really taste authentic, not to mention delicious.

1 pound large shrimp, peeled and
   deveined
1 (10-ounce) package frozen chopped
   spinach, thawed and squeezed dry
½ cup chopped scallions
2 teaspoons Asian chili paste with garlic
2 teaspoons grated fresh ginger
1 teaspoon sesame oil
2 packets artificial sweetener
   (Splenda or Truvia)
2 teaspoons dry sherry
2 teaspoons light soy sauce
½ pound (8 large) cabbage leaves,
   steamed until soft
2 cups water

Asian dipping sauce
(makes approximately 1 cup):

¾ cup light soy sauce
¼ cup rice vinegar
2 teaspoons red pepper flakes, or to taste
1 teaspoon sesame oil
Brown-sugar artificial sweetener
   (1 teaspoon equivalent)

1. In a food processor, pulse shrimp to a coarse paste.
2. In a bowl, mix shrimp with spinach, scallions, chili paste, ginger, sesame oil, sweetener, sherry, and soy sauce until well combined.
3. *To make dumplings:* Lay one cabbage leaf on a flat surface, such as a countertop or cutting board. Cut out and discard rib from center of leaf. In middle of leaf half, mound 1 heaping tablespoon of shrimp mixture. Fold top and bottom of leaf over filling, then fold in sides of leaf (you may need a toothpick to hold closed). Repeat process until all leaves are filled.
4. In a large pot or lidded skillet, bring water to a boil. Place a steamer insert in pot and arrange dumplings in steamer. Cover and steam for 8 to 10 minutes.
5. *To make sauce:* In a small bowl, combine all dipping sauce ingredients.

Makes 4 servings (16 dumplings)

SERVING GUIDELINES

➤ **FOR GASTRIC SLEEVE AND BYPASS:**
   Week 1: Liquid diet.
   Weeks 2–4: Puree 2 steamed dumplings with 2
      tablespoons sauce.
   Weeks 5+: Serve 2–4 steamed dumplings as is
      with sauce.

➤ **FOR BPD-DS:**
   Week 1: Liquid diet.
   Weeks 2–3: Puree 2 steamed dumplings with 2
      tablespoons sauce.
   Weeks 4+: Serve 3–4 steamed dumplings with
      sauce.

➤ **FOR LAP-BAND:**
   Week 1: Liquid diet.
   Weeks 2–4: Puree 2 steamed dumplings with 2
      tablespoons sauce.
   Weeks 5+: Serve 2–4 steamed dumplings as is
      with sauce.

➤ **FOR OTHERS:**
   Serve 4 steamed dumplings with sauce.

Dumplings:

Calories: 176, **Protein:** 26 g, **Fat:** 3 g, **Carbohydrates:** 9 g, **Cholesterol:** 172 mg, **Fiber:** 5 g, **Sodium:** 365 mg

Dipping Sauce (2 tablespoons):

Calories: 15, **Protein:** 1 g, **Fat:** 0 g, **Carbohydrates:** 2 g, **Cholesterol:** 0 mg, **Fiber:** 0 g, **Sodium:** 407 mg

Zucchini Pasta with Shrimp

Think you're going to miss real pasta? Guess again. Just try this zasta (zucchini pasta) in a creamy, garlicky sauce with juicy shrimp.

Pasta:
Olive oil cooking spray

¼ cup water

2 large zucchini, peeled and spiralized or cut into long, thin strips

Shrimp and sauce:
1 cup low-fat ricotta cheese

4 large garlic cloves, minced

1 (14.5-ounce) can low-sodium diced tomatoes

½ cup bottled clam juice

1 tablespoon dried basil

1 teaspoon dried oregano

1 pound fresh, large shrimp, peeled and cleaned

1. Coat a large lidded skillet with cooking spray and heat over medium-high heat until it shimmers. Add water and zucchini pasta and cook, stirring, for 3 to 5 minutes. Remove from pan.

2. In a food processor or blender, puree ricotta cheese until smooth.

3. Dry and re-spray skillet. Over medium heat, sauté garlic until soft, add tomatoes, clam juice, and spices and cook, stirring, for 5 minutes.

4. Lower heat and stir in shrimp. Cover pan and cook until shrimp are pink and cooked through, 3 to 5 minutes. Stir in pureed ricotta cheese and heat for 2 minutes. Pour over zasta.

Makes 4 servings

SERVING GUIDELINES

▶ **FOR GASTRIC SLEEVE AND BYPASS:**
Week 1: Liquid diet.
Weeks 2–3: Puree 1–2 ounces cooked shrimp and sauce with 1 ounce zasta.
Weeks 4–7: Chop 1–2 ounces cooked shrimp and sauce with 1 ounce zasta.
Weeks 8+: Serve 2–4 ounces cooked shrimp with sauce and 1 ounce zasta.

▶ **FOR BPD-DS:**
Week 1: Liquid diet.
Weeks 2–3: Puree 1–2 ounces cooked shrimp and sauce with 1 ounce zasta.
Weeks 4–7: Chop 1–2 ounces cooked shrimp and sauce with 1 ounce zasta.
Weeks 8+: Serve 2–4 ounces cooked shrimp with sauce and 1 ounce zasta.

▶ **FOR LAP-BAND:**
Week 1: Liquid diet.
Weeks 2–3: Puree 1–2 ounces cooked shrimp and sauce with 1 ounce zasta.
Weeks 4–7: Chop 1–2 ounces cooked shrimp and sauce with 1 ounce zasta.
Weeks 8+: Serve 2–4 ounces cooked shrimp with sauce and 1 ounce zasta.

▶ **FOR OTHERS:**
Serve 4–6 cooked shrimp with sauce and 2–4 ounces zasta.

Calories: 235, **Protein:** 31 g, **Fat:** 5 g, **Carbohydrates:** 15 g, **Cholesterol:** 15 mg, **Fiber:** 3 g, **Sodium:** 213 mg

Asian Marinated Scallops

This is a light way to treat the delicate flavor of scallops—a lively Chinese-inspired marinade with citrus and ginger.

Marinade:

½ cup low-sodium soy sauce
¼ teaspoon fresh lime juice
¼ teaspoon fresh orange juice
¼ teaspoon fresh lemon juice
Brown-sugar artificial sweetener
   (1½ teaspoons equivalent)
1 tablespoon grated fresh ginger
1 teaspoon Asian sesame oil

1 pound (about 12) sea scallops
Cooking spray

1. In a wide shallow bowl, combine marinade ingredients and mix well.
2. Add scallops and marinate at room temperature for 5 minutes (2½ minutes on each side). Do not marinate for any longer or scallops will turn soft. Reserving marinade, transfer scallops to a plate.
3. Heat cooking spray in a large nonstick skillet over medium-high heat until hot but not smoking. Sauté scallops for 2 minutes on each side until golden brown and just cooked through. Transfer to a plate.
4. Add marinade to skillet and boil over medium-high heat until reduced to about half (¼ cup).

Makes 4 servings

SERVING GUIDELINES

► **FOR GASTRIC SLEEVE AND BYPASS:**
   Week 1: Liquid diet.
   Weeks 2–4: Puree 2 cooked scallops with 1 tablespoon sauce.
   Weeks 5–7: Chop 2 cooked scallops and top with sauce.
   Weeks 8+: Serve 2–3 cooked scallops with sauce.

► **FOR BPD-DS:**
   Week 1: Liquid diet.
   Weeks 2–3: Puree 2 cooked scallops with 1 tablespoon sauce.
   Weeks 4+: Serve 2–3 cooked scallops with sauce.

► **FOR LAP-BAND:**
   Week 1: Liquid diet.
   Weeks 2–4: Puree 2 cooked scallops with 1 tablespoon sauce.
   Weeks 5–7: Chop 2 cooked scallops and top with sauce.
   Weeks 8+: Serve 2–3 cooked scallops with sauce.

► **FOR OTHERS:**
   Serve 3 cooked scallops with sauce.

Calories: 146, **Protein:** 22 g, **Fat:** 2 g, **Carbohydrates:** 7 g, **Cholesterol:** 37 mg, **Fiber:** 0 g, **Sodium:** 1,267 mg

Coquilles Saint-Jacques

This updated classic is proof that you don't need cream or butter to make an incredibly rich-tasting dish. If you want to be really fancy, serve the scallops mounded in scallop shells.

Butter-flavored cooking spray
3 pinches crumbled saffron
1 pound (about 12) sea scallops, patted dry, tough side muscle removed (if necessary)
¼ cup minced shallots
1 tablespoon white wine
1 tablespoon dry vermouth
½ cup bottled clam juice
½ cup evaporated skim milk

1. Coat a large nonstick skillet with cooking spray. Sprinkle pan with a pinch of saffron and heat over medium-high heat until moderately hot but not smoking.
2. Add scallops in a single layer and cook them undisturbed for 2 minutes on each side, or until golden and just cooked through. Remove scallops and keep warm.
3. Re-spray pan, sprinkle with remaining saffron, and lower heat to low. Add shallots, stirring until soft.
4. Add wine and vermouth to deglaze skillet, scraping up any browned bits. Increase heat to medium-high, add clam juice, and boil until liquid is reduced by half.
5. Add evaporated milk and any scallop juices that have accumulated. Lower heat and simmer until reduced to a thickened, creamy consistency. Stir in scallops.

Makes 4 servings

SERVING GUIDELINES

▶ **FOR GASTRIC SLEEVE AND BYPASS:**
Week 1: Liquid diet.
Weeks 2–4: Puree 2 cooked scallops with 2 tablespoons sauce.
Weeks 5–7: Chop 2 cooked scallops and top with sauce.
Weeks 8+: Serve 2–3 cooked scallops with sauce.

▶ **FOR BPD-DS:**
Week 1: Liquid diet.
Weeks 2–3: Puree 2 cooked scallops with 2 tablespoons sauce.
Weeks 4+: Serve 2–3 cooked scallops with sauce.

▶ **FOR LAP-BAND:**
Week 1: Liquid diet.
Weeks 2–4: Puree 2 cooked scallops with 2 tablespoons sauce.
Weeks 5–7: Chop 2 cooked scallops and top with sauce.
Weeks 8+: Serve 2–3 cooked scallops with sauce.

▶ **FOR OTHERS:**
Serve 3 cooked scallops with sauce.

Calories: 142, **Protein:** 22 g, **Fat:** 1 g, **Carbohydrates:** 9 g, **Cholesterol:** 37 mg, **Fiber:** 0 g, **Sodium:** 261 mg

Scallops Piquant

An easy yet elegant way to prepare scallops. Reducing the mustard-wine sauce gives it a lush, creamy consistency.

Olive oil cooking spray
1 pound (about 12) sea scallops, patted dry, tough side muscle removed (if necessary)
½ cup minced shallots
½ cup white wine
½ cup water
¼ cup Dijon mustard

1. Heat cooking spray in a large nonstick skillet over medium-high heat until hot but not smoking. Sauté scallops for 1 to 2 minutes on each side (depending on size), or until golden and just cooked through. Remove from pan and keep warm.
2. Re-spray skillet and cook shallots over medium heat, stirring, for 1 minute until softened.
3. Add wine and boil, then cook, scraping up any browned bits, for 1 minute. Stir in water and mustard, lower heat, and simmer for 7 to 8 minutes, or until liquid is reduced to about ¾ cup.

Makes 4 servings

SERVING GUIDELINES

➤ **FOR GASTRIC SLEEVE AND BYPASS:**
   Week 1: Liquid diet.
   Weeks 2–4: Puree 3 cooked scallop halves with 2 tablespoons sauce.
   Weeks 5–7: Chop 3 cooked scallop halves and top with sauce.
   Weeks 8+: Serve 3–6 cooked scallop halves with sauce.

➤ **FOR BPD-DS:**
   Week 1: Liquid diet.
   Weeks 2–3: Puree 3 cooked scallop halves with 2 tablespoons sauce.
   Weeks 4+: Serve 3 cooked scallop halves with sauce.

➤ **FOR LAP-BAND:**
   Week 1: Liquid diet.
   Weeks 2–4: Puree 3 cooked scallop halves with 2 tablespoons sauce.
   Weeks 5–7: Chop 3 cooked scallop halves and top with sauce.
   Weeks 8+: Serve 6 cooked scallop halves with sauce.

➤ **FOR OTHERS:**
   Serve 6 cooked scallop halves with sauce.

Calories: 154, **Protein:** 21 g, **Fat:** 2 g, **Carbohydrates:** 8 g, **Cholesterol:** 38 mg, **Fiber:** 0 g, **Sodium:** 272 mg

Scallops Provençale

This luscious classic dish is full of the bright summery flavors of fresh basil and ripe tomatoes.

1 pound (about 12) large sea scallops, patted dry, tough side muscle removed (if necessary)
Olive oil cooking spray
4 garlic cloves, thinly sliced
1½ cups diced seeded fresh tomatoes
⅛ teaspoon dried thyme
¼ cup shredded fresh basil
½ cup dry white wine

1. Slice scallops in half horizontally.
2. In a nonstick skillet large enough to hold scallops in one layer, heat cooking spray over medium-high heat until it is hot but not smoking. Sear scallops for 1 to 2 minutes on each side, or until they are golden brown and just cooked through. Use a slotted spoon to transfer scallops to a platter and cover loosely to keep warm.
3. Re-spray pan and cook garlic over moderate heat, stirring until it is lightly browned.
4. Add tomatoes, thyme, and basil and cook, stirring, for 1 minute.
5. Add wine and cook, stirring, for 1 minute. Lower heat and simmer for about 5 minutes, or until tomatoes are soft and sauce is slightly thickened.

Makes 4 servings

SERVING GUIDELINES

► **FOR GASTRIC SLEEVE AND BYPASS:**
Week 1: Liquid diet.
Weeks 2–4: Puree 3 cooked scallop halves with 2 tablespoons sauce.
Weeks 5–7: Chop 3 cooked scallop halves and top with sauce.
Weeks 8+: Serve 3–6 cooked scallop halves with sauce.

► **FOR BPD-DS:**
Week 1: Liquid diet.
Weeks 2–3: Puree 3 cooked scallop halves with 2 tablespoons sauce.
Weeks 4+: Serve 3–6 cooked scallop halves with sauce.

► **FOR LAP-BAND:**
Week 1: Liquid diet.
Weeks 2–4: Puree 3 cooked scallop halves with 2 tablespoons sauce.
Weeks 5–7: Chop 3 cooked scallop halves and top with sauce.
Weeks 8+: Serve 3–6 cooked scallop halves with sauce.

► **FOR OTHERS:**
Serve 6 cooked scallop halves with sauce.

Calories: 140, **Protein:** 20 g, **Fat:** 1 g, **Carbohydrates:** 7 g, **Cholesterol:** 37 mg, **Fiber:** 1 g, **Sodium:** 191 mg

Scallops with White Wine and Garlic

This dish couldn't be simpler to make, and the garlic seems to intensify the sweet scallop flavor.

1 pound (about 12) sea scallops, patted dry, tough side muscle removed (if necessary)

Olive oil cooking spray

8 garlic cloves, minced

¾ cup white wine

¼ cup minced fresh parsley, or 3 tablespoons dried

1. Slice scallops in half horizontally.
2. In a nonstick skillet large enough to hold all scallops in one layer, heat cooking spray over medium-high heat until hot but not smoking. Add scallops, sprinkle with garlic, and brown well on one side, 2 to 3 minutes.
3. Turn scallops and brown well on other side (garlic should get brown and crunchy). Remove scallops from pan and keep warm.
4. Deglaze pan with white wine, scraping up any browned bits and garlic.
5. Add parsley and simmer, uncovered, for 5 minutes.

Makes 4 servings

SERVING GUIDELINES

▸ **FOR GASTRIC SLEEVE AND BYPASS:**
Week 1: Liquid diet.
Weeks 2–4: Puree 3 cooked scallop halves with 2 tablespoons sauce.
Weeks 5–7: Chop 3 cooked scallop halves and top with sauce.
Weeks 8+: Serve 3–6 cooked scallop halves with sauce.

▸ **FOR BPD-DS:**
Week 1: Liquid diet.
Weeks 2–3: Puree 3 cooked scallop halves with 2 tablespoons sauce.
Weeks 4+: Serve 3–6 cooked scallop halves with sauce.

▸ **FOR LAP-BAND:**
Week 1: Liquid diet.
Weeks 2–4: Puree 3 cooked scallop halves with 2 tablespoons sauce.
Weeks 5–7: Chop 3 cooked scallop halves and top with sauce.
Weeks 8+: Serve 3–6 cooked scallop halves with sauce.

▸ **FOR OTHERS:**
Serve 6 cooked scallop halves with sauce.

Calories: 140, **Protein:** 20 g, **Fat:** 1 g, **Carbohydrates:** 5 g, **Cholesterol:** 37 mg, **Fiber:** 0 g, **Sodium:** 188 mg

The Most Versatile Vegetable Recipe Ever

It works for every meal and you make it in the microwave.

1 large sweet onion, peeled and chopped

6 large mushrooms, rinsed and thinly sliced

1 red, yellow, or orange bell pepper, seeded and chopped

20 grape or cherry tomatoes, cut in half

2 teaspoons unsalted butter

2 teaspoons savory spice blend (steak rub, Tex-Mex, fines herbes, etc.)

1 Hass avocado, peeled, seeded, and diced

1. Combine all ingredients, except avocado, in a microwaveable bowl and cover tightly with plastic wrap.
2. Microwave on HIGH for 6 minutes.
3. Remove from microwave, let stand for 2 minutes, then stir in avocado.

Now here's what I mean about versatile:

BREAKFAST: Fold into an omelet with one slice low-fat Swiss cheese or stir into scrambled eggs with 2 tablespoons shredded low-fat Cheddar.

LUNCH: Mix ½ cup vegetable recipe with ½ cup low-fat or fat-free cottage cheese or ricotta cheese, or mix ½ cup vegetable recipe with ½ cup canned tuna or salmon, or for a delicious soup, just add the entire vegetable recipe to 3 cups low-sodium beef, chicken, or vegetable broth with a can of drained and rinsed beans.

DINNER: Make it Italian: Brown 1 pound lean ground turkey or beef with 1 teaspoon minced garlic; drain off fat. Make vegetable recipe with an Italian savory spice blend (basil, oregano, Parmesan) and mix with the meat.

Make it Indian: Make vegetable recipe with a savory curry spice blend and mix it with 1 pound cooked shredded chicken or lamb, or keep it vegetarian mixed with a can of low-sodium lentils, drained and rinsed.

Make it Mexican: Brown 1 pound lean ground turkey or beef and drain. Add ½ seeded and diced fresh chile pepper and ¼ cup minced fresh cilantro. Make vegetable recipe with a Mexican spice blend, mix with the meat, and top with fat-free sour cream or low-fat shredded Cheddar. Or keep it vegetarian and substitute a can of low-sodium red or black beans, drained and rinsed, for the meat.

SNACK OR APPETIZER: Mix vegetable recipe with 8 ounces fat-free cream cheese and serve with raw vegetables or chunks of turkey pepperoni or turkey salami.

Makes 4 servings

➤ **Note:** The nutritional analysis was computed for the veggie recipe alone. If you want to make any of the other suggestions, the nutritional analysis will change. Also, Meredith recommends that you not eat the basic veggie recipe alone until after Week 5.

SERVING GUIDELINES *(FOR VEGGIE RECIPE ALONE)*

➤ **FOR GASTRIC SLEEVE AND BYPASS:**
Week 1: Liquid diet.
Weeks 2–5: Not recommended.
Weeks 6+: Serve 2 ounces of vegetables as a side dish.

➤ **FOR BPD-DS:**
Week 1: Liquid diet.
Weeks 2–5: Not recommended.
Weeks 6+: Serve 2 ounces of vegetables as a side dish.

➤ **FOR LAP-BAND:**
Week 1: Liquid diet.
Weeks 2–5: Not recommended.
Weeks 6+: Serve 2 ounces of vegetables as a side dish.

➤ **FOR OTHERS:**
Serve 4 ounces of vegetables as a side dish.

Calories: 152, **Protein:** 2 g, **Fat:** 6 g, **Carbohydrates:** 19 g, **Cholesterol:** 2 mg, **Fiber:** 4 g, **Sodium:** 27 mg

Vegetarian Bean Chili

I developed this recipe for those readers who requested vegetarian dishes and "not-so-fancy" dishes. You can make it as spicy as you like—just add more jalapeños and chili powder—neither one will add fat or carbs.

Olive oil cooking spray
1 medium carrot, peeled and diced
1 medium yellow onion, peeled and diced
2 garlic cloves, minced
1 medium red, yellow, or orange bell
  pepper, seeded and diced
1 jalapeño pepper, ribs and seeds
  removed, minced
3 celery stalks, diced
½ teaspoon dried oregano
1 teaspoon ground cumin
1 teaspoon chili powder
1 (15.5-ounce) can low-sodium diced
  tomatoes with chiles
1 (15.5-ounce) can low-sodium tomato
  sauce
1 cup low-sodium vegetable broth
1 (15.5-ounce) can low-sodium kidney
  beans, drained and rinsed
1 (15.5-ounce) can low-sodium pinto
  beans, drained and rinsed
1 (15.5-ounce) can low-sodium black
  beans, drained and rinsed
2 medium zucchini, diced
Salt to taste

1. Coat a large lidded pot with cooking spray and heat over medium-high heat until hot.
2. Add carrot, onion, garlic, bell pepper, jalapeño, and celery and cook, stirring, for 7 to 9 minutes, or until onion turns golden brown.
3. Stir in oregano, cumin, and chili powder and cook for 2 minutes.
4. Pour in diced tomatoes, tomato sauce, and broth and bring to a boil, then lower heat to low and simmer, stirring, for 30 minutes.
5. Stir in beans and zucchini, cover pot, and simmer for 45 minutes to 1 hour, or until thick (if too soupy, increase heat and cook, uncovered, stirring, for 15 minutes more).
6. Add salt to taste.

Makes 8 to 12 servings; can be frozen

➤ **Note:** I don't own a slow cooker but I'm sure that you can cook this recipe in one.

SERVING GUIDELINES

➤ **FOR GASTRIC SLEEVE AND BYPASS:**
   Week 1: Liquid diet.
   Weeks 2–7: Puree 2 ounces chili.
   Weeks 8+: Serve 2–4 ounces chili.

➤ **FOR BPD-DS:**
   Week 1: Liquid diet.
   Weeks 2–7: Puree 2 ounces chili.
   Weeks 8+: Serve 2–4 ounces chili.

➤ **FOR LAP-BAND:**
   Week 1: Liquid diet.
   Weeks 2–7: Puree 2 ounces chili.
   Weeks 8+: Serve 2–4 ounces chili.

➤ **FOR OTHERS:**
   Serve 1 cup chili.

Calories: 204, **Protein:** 12 g, **Fat:** 1 g, **Carbohydrates:** 38 g, **Cholesterol:** 0 mg, **Fiber:** 13 g, **Sodium:** 677 mg

Fresh Veggie Burgers

Even though I'm a carnivore, this veggie burger tastes good to me—plus, it really beats out those processed ones you get in the supermarket. Instead of ketchup, why not top it with our Garlic Sauce (page 186), Quick Tomato Sauce (page 193) or Sauce Piperade (page 194)?

1 (15-ounce) can low-sodium pinto beans, drained and rinsed
Cooking spray
1 small white or yellow onion, diced small
1 garlic clove, minced
3 green onions or scallions, thinly sliced
1 teaspoon cumin
¾ cup diced fresh mushrooms
1 teaspoon dried parsley
Salt and pepper to taste

1. In a bowl, mash pinto beans with a fork or potato masher until smooth. Or pulse in a food processor until smooth.
2. Spray a skillet with cooking spray. Heat over medium heat until it shimmers.
3. Sauté onion and garlic for 3 to 5 minutes, or until soft.
4. Add green onions, cumin, mushrooms, and parsley and cook, stirring occasionally, for 5 minutes. Remove from pan.
5. Mix mashed beans with mushroom mixture and salt and pepper to taste, and form into 1-inch-thick patties.
6. Wipe out skillet, re-spray, and sauté patties for 3 to 4 minutes on each side, or until cooked through.

Makes 4 servings

SERVING GUIDELINES

▶ **FOR GASTRIC SLEEVE AND BYPASS:**
   Week 1: Liquid diet.
   Weeks 2–4: Puree ½ cooked burger with 2 tablespoons sauce.
   Weeks 5–7: Chop ½ cooked burger and top with 2 tablespoons sauce.
   Weeks 8+: Serve ½–1 cooked burger with 2 tablespoons sauce.

▶ **FOR BPD-DS:**
   Week 1: Liquid diet.
   Weeks 2–4: Puree ½ cooked burger with 2 tablespoons sauce.
   Weeks 5–7: Chop ½ cooked burger and top with 2 tablespoons sauce.
   Weeks 8+: Serve ½–1 cooked burger with 2 tablespoons sauce.

▶ **FOR LAP-BAND:**
   Week 1: Liquid diet.
   Weeks 2–4: Puree ½ cooked burger with 2 tablespoons sauce.
   Weeks 5–7: Chop ½ cooked burger and top with 2 tablespoons sauce.
   Weeks 8+: Serve ½–1 cooked burger with 2 tablespoons sauce.

▶ **FOR OTHERS:**
   Serve 1 cooked burger with 2 tablespoons sauce.

Calories: 122, **Protein:** 8 g, **Fat:** 0 g, **Carbohydrates:** 21 g, **Cholesterol:** 0 mg, **Fiber:** 8 g, **Sodium:** 119 mg

Vegetarian Portobello Mushroom and Butter Bean Stew

If you've been looking for a delicious vegetarian dish that's not just the same old–same old, try this one. The portobello mushrooms make it rich and hearty.

Olive oil cooking spray
1 large onion, sliced
4 large portobello mushroom caps, thickly sliced
3 garlic cloves, minced
2 (14.5-ounce) cans butter beans or lima beans, drained and rinsed
2 teaspoons dried thyme
1 teaspoon lemon-pepper
1 (28-ounce) can low-sodium whole peeled tomatoes
1½ cups low-sodium vegetable broth
1 tablespoon Marmite or concentrated vegetarian broth

1. In a large pot, heat olive oil spray over medium-high heat until it shimmers.
2. Add onion, mushrooms, and garlic. Cover and cook until onion is translucent and mushrooms begin to give up their liquid, 7 to 10 minutes.
3. Stir in beans, thyme, and lemon-pepper.
4. Add tomatoes and smash them with back of a spoon. Stir in broth and Marmite or concentrate.
5. Cover and simmer over low heat for 2 hours, stirring occasionally, until thick and most of liquid has evaporated.

Makes 4 servings

SERVING GUIDELINES

➤ **FOR GASTRIC SLEEVE AND BYPASS:**
 Week 1: Liquid diet.
 Weeks 2–3: Puree 2 ounces stew.
 Weeks 4–7: Chop 2 ounces stew.
 Weeks 8+: Serve 2–4 ounces stew.

➤ **FOR BPD-DS:**
 Week 1: Liquid diet.
 Weeks 2–3: Puree 2 ounces stew.
 Weeks 4+: Serve 2–4 ounces stew.

➤ **FOR LAP-BAND:**
 Week 1: Liquid diet.
 Weeks 2–3: Puree 2 ounces stew.
 Weeks 4–7: Chop 2 ounces stew.
 Weeks 8+: Serve 2–4 ounces stew.

➤ **FOR OTHERS:**
 Serve 4–8 ounces stew.

Calories: 325, **Protein:** 19 g, **Fat:** 1 g, **Carbohydrates:** 63 g, **Cholesterol:** 0 mg, **Fiber:** 16 g, **Sodium:** 215 mg

Orange-Ginger Tofu

This is a light and refreshing Chinese-influenced recipe that's just as tasty served hot as it is cold. If you want a truly vegetarian dish, you can substitute vegetable broth for the chicken broth, but remember, it may change the nutritional analysis numbers.

1 tablespoon orange zest
½ cup fresh orange juice
1 cup fat-free, low-sodium chicken broth
1 tablespoon dry sherry
Brown-sugar artificial sweetener
  (1 teaspoon equivalent)
1 tablespoon sesame oil
Cooking spray
1 tablespoon minced fresh ginger
2 large garlic cloves, minced
2 large leeks, washed thoroughly and
  sliced thinly (about 1½ cups)
1 pound firm tofu, drained and cubed

1. Combine orange zest, juice, chicken broth, sherry, sweetener, and sesame oil in a small bowl and set aside.
2. Heat cooking spray in a medium nonstick skillet over medium-high heat until hot but not smoking. Stir-fry ginger and garlic for 30 seconds. Add leeks and stir-fry for 3 minutes.
3. Add tofu and stir-fry for 4 minutes. Remove tofu-vegetable mixture from pan.
4. Pour orange juice mixture into pan, bring to a boil, lower heat, and cook for 10 minutes, or until reduced by half.
5. Stir in tofu-vegetable mixture and simmer for 1 minute.

Makes 4 servings

SERVING GUIDELINES

▶ **FOR GASTRIC SLEEVE AND BYPASS:**
  Week 1: Liquid diet.
  Weeks 2–4: Puree ¼–½ cup cooked tofu mixture until smooth.
  Weeks 5–7: Chop ¼–½ cup cooked tofu mixture.
  Weeks 8+: Serve ½–¾ cup cooked tofu mixture as is.

▶ **FOR BPD-DS:**
  Week 1: Liquid diet.
  Weeks 2–3: Puree ¼–½ cup cooked tofu mixture until smooth.
  Weeks 4+: Serve ½–1 cup cooked tofu mixture as is.

▶ **FOR LAP-BAND:**
  Week 1: Liquid diet.
  Weeks 2–4: Puree ¼–½ cup cooked tofu mixture until smooth.
  Weeks 5–7: Chop ¼–½ cup cooked tofu mixture.
  Weeks 8+: Serve ½–¾ cup cooked tofu mixture as is.

▶ **FOR OTHERS:**
  Serve 1 cup cooked tofu mixture as is.

Calories: 250, **Protein:** 20 g, **Fat:** 14 g, **Carbohydrates:** 14 g, **Cholesterol:** 0 mg, **Fiber:** 3 g, **Sodium:** 41 mg

Tofu and Vegetable Curry

This is a classic vegetable curry—we just added some tofu for protein. If you like your curry hotter, you can increase the curry paste or throw in some minced hot peppers.

1 cup light unsweetened coconut milk

3 packets artificial sweetener
  (Splenda or Truvia)

2 tablespoons light soy sauce

1½ tablespoons grated fresh ginger

2 garlic cloves, minced

1 teaspoon green curry paste

Butter-flavored cooking spray

1 pound extra-firm tofu, drained and cut
  into 1-inch cubes

1 cup seeded and thinly sliced red bell
  pepper

4 cups shredded cabbage

1 cup fat-free, low-sodium vegetable broth

1 cup chopped scallions

3 tablespoons chopped fresh cilantro

1. In a small bowl, combine coconut milk, sweetener, soy sauce, ginger, garlic, and curry paste.

2. In a large nonstick lidded skillet, heat cooking spray over medium heat until hot but not smoking. Add tofu and sauté, stirring occasionally, for 10 minutes, or until golden brown. Remove from pan and keep warm.

3. Add bell pepper to pan and sauté for 1 minute. Add cabbage and broth, lower heat, cover, and simmer for 15 minutes.

4. Stir in coconut milk mixture, scallions, cilantro, and tofu and cook for 2 minutes.

Makes 4 servings

SERVING GUIDELINES

➤ **FOR GASTRIC SLEEVE AND BYPASS:**
  Week 1: Liquid diet.
  Weeks 2–4: Puree ¼–½ cup cooked curry until smooth.
  Weeks 5–7: Chop ¼–½ cup cooked curry.
  Weeks 8+: Serve ½–¾ cup cooked curry as is.

➤ **FOR BPD-DS:**
  Week 1: Liquid diet.
  Weeks 2–3: Puree ¼–½ cup cooked curry until smooth.
  Weeks 4+: Serve ½–1 cup cooked curry as is.

➤ **FOR LAP-BAND:**
  Week 1: Liquid diet.
  Weeks 2–4: Puree ¼–½ cup cooked curry until smooth.
  Weeks 5–7: Chop ¼–½ cup cooked curry.
  Weeks 8+: Serve ½–¾ cup cooked curry as is.

➤ **FOR OTHERS:**
  Serve 1 cup cooked curry as is.

Calories: 273, **Protein:** 21 g, **Fat:** 15 g, **Carbohydrates:** 18 g, **Cholesterol:** 0 mg, **Fiber:** 6 g, **Sodium:** 602 mg

Tofu Mexicano

If you're into Tex-Mex flavors, this dish has it all. Here's a serving idea: once you're eating solid food, try spooning each portion onto lettuce leaves and wrapping it like a tortilla.

Canola cooking spray
2 cups chopped onion
1 large garlic clove, minced
½ teaspoon ground cumin
½ teaspoon chili powder
1 pound extra-firm tofu, drained and cubed
1 cup seeded and chopped red or yellow bell pepper
1 small jalapeño pepper, seeded and chopped
1 cup chopped fresh tomatoes
½ cup shredded low-fat Cheddar cheese
Salt and pepper to taste

1. Heat cooking spray in a large nonstick ovenproof skillet over medium-high heat until hot but not smoking. Cook onion, garlic, cumin, and chili powder for 3 minutes, or until onion is softened.
2. Add tofu, bell pepper, jalapeño, and tomatoes and cook for about 3 minutes, or until peppers are softened.
3. Preheat broiler and arrange rack to top position. Sprinkle cheese on top of veggie mixture and place under broiler for 40 seconds, or until cheese melts and becomes bubbly. Add salt and pepper to taste.

Makes 4 servings

SERVING GUIDELINES

► **FOR GASTRIC SLEEVE AND BYPASS:**
  Week 1: Liquid diet.
  Weeks 2–4: Puree ¼–½ cup cooked tofu mixture until smooth.
  Weeks 5–7: Chop ¼–½ cup cooked tofu mixture.
  Weeks 8+: Serve ½–¾ cup cooked tofu mixture as is.

► **FOR BPD-DS:**
  Week 1: Liquid diet.
  Weeks 2–3: Puree ¼–½ cup cooked tofu mixture until smooth.
  Weeks 4+: Serve ½–1 cup cooked tofu mixture as is.

► **FOR LAP-BAND:**
  Week 1: Liquid diet.
  Weeks 2–4: Puree ¼–½ cup cooked tofu mixture until smooth.
  Weeks 5–7: Chop ¼–½ cup cooked tofu mixture.
  Weeks 8+: Serve ½–¾ cup cooked tofu mixture as is.

► **FOR OTHERS:**
  Serve 1 cup cooked tofu mixture as is.

Calories: 309, **Protein:** 27 g, **Fat:** 16 g, **Carbohydrates:** 17 g, **Cholesterol:** 20 mg, **Fiber:** 6 g, **Sodium:** 267 mg

Tofu Tikka

Instead of making the usual tikka with chicken, we decided to substitute tofu. When the tofu is marinated, it really takes on all the spice and flavors, so it seems to explode in your mouth.

1 large garlic clove, chopped
½ teaspoon grated fresh ginger
½ small red chile pepper, seeded
½ teaspoon ground cumin
½ teaspoon ground coriander
½ teaspoon ground turmeric
½ teaspoon garam masala
1 cup plain, fat-free yogurt
2 tablespoons fresh lime juice
1 pound extra-firm tofu, drained and quartered
Butter-flavored cooking spray
½ cup fat-free, low-sodium vegetable broth

1. In a food processor, combine garlic, ginger, and chile and process until finely chopped. Add cumin, coriander, turmeric, garam masala, yogurt, and lime juice and blend to make a smooth paste.
2. Place yogurt mixture in shallow bowl and add tofu, stirring to coat completely. Cover bowl and chill in refrigerator for at least 4 hours.
3. Twenty minutes before cooking, remove tofu from refrigerator and allow to become room temperature. Remove tofu from marinade and scrape off excess, reserving marinade.
4. Coat a large nonstick skillet with cooking spray and sauté tofu over medium-high heat, turning once or twice, for 15 to 20 minutes, or until nicely browned. Remove tofu from pan and cut into 1-inch cubes.
5. Over medium-low heat, deglaze pan with vegetable broth, scraping up any browned bits. Add reserved marinade and tofu back to pan and simmer for 3 minutes.

Makes 4 servings

SERVING GUIDELINES

▶ **FOR GASTRIC SLEEVE AND BYPASS:**
   Week 1: Liquid diet.
   Weeks 2–4: Puree ¼–½ cup cooked tofu mixture until smooth.
   Weeks 5–7: Chop ¼–½ cup cooked tofu mixture.
   Weeks 8+: Serve ½–¾ cup cooked tofu mixture as is.

▶ **FOR BPD-DS:**
   Week 1: Liquid diet.
   Weeks 2–3: Puree ¼–½ cup cooked tofu mixture until smooth.
   Weeks 4+: Serve ½–1 cup cooked tofu mixture as is.

▶ **FOR LAP-BAND:**
   Week 1: Liquid diet.
   Weeks 2–4: Puree ¼–½ cup cooked tofu mixture until smooth.
   Weeks 5–7: Chop ¼–½ cup cooked tofu mixture.
   Weeks 8+: Serve ½–¾ cup cooked tofu mixture as is.

▶ **FOR OTHERS:**
   Serve 1 cup cooked tofu mixture as is.

Calories: 218, **Protein:** 22 g, **Fat:** 10 g, **Carbohydrates:** 13 g, **Cholesterol:** 2 mg, **Fiber:** 3 g, **Sodium:** 205 mg

Sweet Indulgences

Desserts and beverages that taste too good to be true—but they are

SINCE WE DESIGNED this cookbook to be used not just in those first weeks after surgery, but for the months and years after, we knew that we had to include some really great sweets. Let's face it: you can deny your sweet cravings for a while, but not for the rest of your life.

Can you really have desserts? Yes, if they are low-fat, high-protein desserts like the recipes we provide you with here, which are made with no added sugars. They are so delicious even your "others" will enjoy them.

You might be wondering, now that you have to eat so much less, if you will even have room for dessert after a meal. That's a valid concern. You might not be able to eat these dishes directly after a meal, but your nutritionist has probably told you that you can eat one or two healthy snacks during the day. These recipes make perfect snacks—for example, Strawberry Ricotta Whip (page 176) or one of our fresh fruit-and-yogurt smoothies. We've even included a delicious low-fat hot chocolate.

So go ahead, indulge. After all, your surgery didn't remove your sweet tooth.

Note: The nutritional analyses are based on an average portion size (*Others'* portions).

Basic Cheesecake

This is a light, almost fluffy cheesecake that literally melts in your mouth.

1 (8-ounce) container fat-free
   cream cheese
½ pound silken tofu
½ cup egg substitute
6 packets artificial sweetener
   (Splenda or Truvia)
½ teaspoon vanilla extract
¼ teaspoon almond extract
6 tablespoons egg white substitute
¼ teaspoon cream of tartar
Butter-flavored cooking spray

1. Preheat oven to 350°F.
2. In a large bowl, using an electric mixer, beat together cream cheese, tofu, egg substitute, sweetener, vanilla, and almond extract until smooth and creamy.
3. In a small bowl, using an electric mixer, whip egg white substitute with cream of tartar until it forms stiff peaks.
4. Gently fold whipped egg whites into cream cheese mixture.
5. Coat a 8-inch square cake pan with cooking spray and pour in batter. Place cake pan into a baking pan and pour hot water into baking pan until it reaches halfway up sides of cake pan. Place in oven and bake for 30 minutes.
6. Remove from oven, let cool, then refrigerate for at least 4 hours.

Makes 8 servings

► **Hint:** You can serve this cheesecake alone or topped with our Raspberry Sauce (page 204) or Papaya Sauce (page 206).

SERVING GUIDELINES

► **FOR GASTRIC SLEEVE AND BYPASS:**
   Week 1: Liquid diet.
   Weeks 2+: Serve ½ slice cheesecake.

► **FOR BPD-DS:**
   Week 1: Liquid diet.
   Weeks 2+: Serve ½–1 slice cheesecake.

► **FOR LAP-BAND:**
   Week 1: Liquid diet.
   Weeks 2+: Serve ½ slice cheesecake.

► **FOR OTHERS:**
   Serve 1 slice cheesecake.

Calories: 59, **Protein:** 8 g, **Fat:** 1 g, **Carbohydrates:** 4 g, **Cholesterol:** 5 mg, **Fiber:** 0 g, **Sodium:** 186 mg

Minted Cheesecake with Strawberry Sauce

This cheesecake tastes like summer, thanks to the fresh mint leaves.

Cheesecake:
6 ounces fat-free cream cheese, softened
½ cup fat-free ricotta cheese
¼ cup fresh mint leaves
5 packets artificial sweetener
 (Splenda or Truvia)
¼ teaspoon vanilla extract

Strawberry Sauce
(makes approximately 1 cup):
1 cup hulled and sliced fresh strawberries
½ cup water
6 packets artificial sweetener
 (Splenda or Truvia)
½ teaspoon balsamic vinegar

1. *To make cheesecake:* Combine all cheesecake ingredients in food processor and puree until smooth.
2. Pour into four 4-ounce ramekins, cover with plastic wrap, and chill in refrigerator for at least 4 hours.
3. *To make sauce:* In a small saucepan, combine all sauce ingredients and bring to a boil. Lower heat and simmer for 10 minutes, stirring occasionally, until strawberries are soft and sauce is slightly thickened.
4. Pour into a container, cover, and chill for at least 4 hours.

Makes 4 servings

SERVING GUIDELINES

► **FOR GASTRIC SLEEVE AND BYPASS:**
 Week 1: Liquid diet.
 Weeks 2+: Serve 2 ounces cheesecake with 2
  tablespoons sauce.

► **FOR BPD-DS:**
 Week 1: Liquid diet.
 Weeks 2+: Serve 2–4 ounces cheesecake with 2
  tablespoons sauce.

► **FOR LAP-BAND:**
 Week 1: Liquid diet.
 Weeks 2+: Serve 2 ounces cheesecake with 2
  tablespoons sauce.

► **FOR OTHERS:**
 Serve 4 ounces cheesecake with sauce.

Cheesecake:

Calories: 76, **Protein:** 11 g, **Fat:** 0 g, **Carbohydrates:** 8 g, **Cholesterol:** 11 mg, **Fiber:** 1 g, **Sodium:** 229 mg

Strawberry Sauce (2 tablespoons):

Calories: 7, **Protein:** 0 g, **Fat:** 0 g, **Carbohydrates:** 2 g, **Cholesterol:** 0 mg, **Fiber:** 1 g, **Sodium:** 5 mg

Strawberry Ricotta Whip

This light, frothy recipe is tangy, creamy, and full of fresh fruit flavor.

2½ cups hulled and quartered fresh strawberries
½ cup fat-free ricotta cheese
½ cup plain, fat-free yogurt
½ teaspoon grated fresh orange zest
½ teaspoon vanilla extract
4 packets artificial sweetener (Splenda or Truvia)
6 tablespoons egg white substitute
½ teaspoon cream of tartar

1. Combine strawberries, ricotta, yogurt, orange zest, vanilla, and sweetener in bowl of a food processor and process until smooth.
2. In a medium bowl, whip egg white substitute and cream of tartar until stiff peaks form.
3. Gently fold beaten egg whites into strawberry mixture. Pour into four small dessert bowls and chill overnight.

Makes 4 servings

SERVING GUIDELINES

▶ **FOR GASTRIC SLEEVE AND BYPASS:**
   Week 1: Liquid diet.
   Weeks 2+: Serve 2 ounces as is.

▶ **FOR LAP-BAND:**
   Week 1: Liquid diet.
   Weeks 2+: Serve 2 ounces as is.

▶ **FOR BPD-DS:**
   Week 1: Liquid diet.
   Weeks 2+: Serve 2–4 ounces as is.

▶ **FOR OTHERS:**
   Serve 4 ounces as is.

Calories: 86, **Protein:** 9 g, **Fat:** 0 g, **Carbohydrates:** 14 g, **Cholesterol:** 4 mg, **Fiber:** 2 g, **Sodium:** 85 mg

Flan

Some call it flan, some call it custard—I call it delicious. This light, low-fat version is surprisingly satisfying to your sweet tooth.

1 (12-ounce) can fat-free evaporated milk
½ teaspoon vanilla extract
8 packets artificial sweetener
   (Splenda or Truvia)
1 large egg
1 large egg yolk

Special equipment:
You'll need six 4-ounce custard cups or
   ramekins for this recipe.

1. Preheat oven to 350°F.
2. Whisk together all ingredients until smooth.
3. Divide mixture equally among six custard cups and place cups in a baking pan filled with 1 inch of hot water. Cover baking pan loosely with a sheet of aluminum foil and bake in middle of oven until flan is set but still trembles slightly, 35 to 40 minutes.
4. Remove cups from baking dish and let cool on rack. Then, place cups in refrigerator and chill, uncovered, at least 2 hours.
5. Serve in cups or unmold by running a knife around edges to loosen and invert onto plates.

Makes 6 servings

► **Hint:** This can be served plain or topped with 2 tablespoons of Papaya Sauce (page 206), Chocolate Sauce (page 203), or Raspberry Sauce (page 204).

SERVING GUIDELINES

► **FOR GASTRIC SLEEVE AND BYPASS:**
   Week 1: Liquid diet.
   Weeks 2+: Serve 2 ounces as is.

► **FOR BPD-DS:**
   Week 1: Liquid diet.
   Weeks 2+: Serve 2–4 ounces as is.

► **FOR LAP-BAND:**
   Week 1: Liquid diet.
   Weeks 2+: Serve 2 ounces as is.

► **FOR OTHERS:**
   Serve 4 ounces as is.

Calories: 73, **Protein:** 6 g, **Fat:** 2 g, **Carbohydrates:** 10 g, **Cholesterol:** 71 mg, **Fiber:** 0 g, **Sodium:** 92 mg

Lemon Soufflé

This tart, frothy dessert is really quite simple to make. The secret is not to open the oven while it's baking and to serve it immediately.

2 large eggs, separated
2 tablespoons grated lemon zest
¼ cup fresh lemon juice
6 packets artificial sweetener
   (Splenda or Truvia)
1 (12-ounce) can fat-free evaporated milk

1. Preheat oven to 350°F.
2. Beat egg whites until stiff.
3. In a separate bowl, mix all other ingredients together and gently fold in egg whites.
4. Pour into a 2-quart casserole or soufflé dish and place dish in a baking pan. Pour hot water into baking pan until it reaches halfway up sides of soufflé dish.
5. Bake for 35 minutes.

Makes 4 servings

SERVING GUIDELINES

► **FOR GASTRIC SLEEVE AND BYPASS:**
   Week 1: Liquid diet.
   Weeks 2+: Serve 2 ounces baked soufflé as is.

► **FOR BPD-DS:**
   Week 1: Liquid diet.
   Weeks 2+: Serve 2–4 ounces baked soufflé as is.

► **FOR LAP-BAND:**
   Week 1: Liquid diet.
   Weeks 2+: Serve 2 ounces baked soufflé as is.

► **FOR OTHERS:**
   Serve 4 ounces baked soufflé as is.

Calories: 118, **Protein:** 9 g, **Fat:** 3 g, **Carbohydrates:** 16 g, **Cholesterol:** 106 mg, **Fiber:** 0 g, **Sodium:** 152 mg

Apricot and Strawberry Smoothie

If you're looking for a healthy, protein-rich snack, fruit smoothies are perfect. This one is fresh and tangy-tasting, and the color is spectacular.

1 small very ripe apricot, pitted and cut into eighths
2 fresh strawberries, hulled and cut into quarters (about ¼ cup)
½ cup plain, fat-free yogurt
¼ cup skim milk
1 packet artificial sweetener (Splenda or Truvia)

1. Place all ingredients in a blender and puree until frothy.

Makes 1 serving

➤ **Variation:** Summer slushy—if your blender can crush ice, add two ice cubes before blending.

SERVING GUIDELINES

➤ **FOR EVERYONE WHO'S HAD BARIATRIC SURGERY:**
Week 1: Liquid diet.
Weeks 2+: Serve as is.

➤ **FOR OTHERS:**
Serve as is.

Calories: 137, **Protein:** 11 g, **Fat:** 0 g, **Carbohydrates:** 23 g, **Cholesterol:** 5 mg, **Fiber:** 2 g, **Sodium:** 159 mg

Minted Summer Smoothie

Cucumber in a smoothie? You'll be amazed at how refreshing it is. We combined it with sweet melon, but you can try other ripe fruit.

½ cup diced ripe honeydew melon
¼ cup peeled, diced cucumber
6 fresh mint leaves
½ cup plain, fat-free yogurt
1 packet artificial sweetener
   (Splenda or Truvia)
2 ice cubes

1. Put all ingredients, except ice cubes, in a blender and puree until smooth.
2. Add ice cubes and blend on high speed for about 30 seconds until chilled.

Makes 1 serving

SERVING GUIDELINES

► **FOR EVERYONE WHO'S HAD BARIATRIC SURGERY:**
   Week 1: Liquid diet.
   Weeks 2+: Serve as is.

► **FOR OTHERS:**
   Serve as is.

Calories: 140, **Protein:** 10 g, **Fat:** 0 g, **Carbohydrates:** 27 g, **Cholesterol:** 3 mg, **Fiber:** 3 g, **Sodium:** 145 mg

Piña Colada Smoothie

Talk about tropical—this smoothie brings back memories of island beaches, hibiscus flowers, and soft breezes. In other words, you'll have a vacation in a glass.

½ cup plain, fat-free yogurt
¼ cup diced fresh pineapple
¼ cup diced fresh mango
2 packets artificial sweetener
  (Splenda or Truvia)
½ teaspoon coconut extract
3 ice cubes

1. Place all ingredients in a blender and puree until frothy.

Serves 1

SERVING GUIDELINES

➤ **FOR EVERYONE WHO'S HAD BARIATRIC SURGERY:**
  Week 1: Liquid diet.
  Weeks 2+: Serve as is.

➤ **FOR OTHERS:**
  Serve as is.

Calories: 133, **Protein:** 8 g, **Fat:** 0 g, **Carbohydrates:** 27 g, **Cholesterol:** 3 mg, **Fiber:** 1 g, **Sodium:** 128 mg

Hot Chocolate

Surprise, surprise—hot chocolate is allowable, as long as it's made like this. Actually, it's a great way to get your daily protein and calcium.

1 tablespoon unsweetened cocoa powder
1 packet artificial sweetener
   (Splenda or Truvia)
1 cup skim milk

1. Mix cocoa and sweetener in a cup or mug.
2. Add ¼ cup milk and stir to make a paste.
3. Heat remaining ¾ cup milk in microwave on HIGH for 45 seconds to 1 minute, or until hot. *For stovetop:* Pour remaining ¾ cup milk into a small saucepan and simmer over low heat for 1 to 2 minutes. Add hot milk to cocoa mixture, stirring until smooth.

Makes 1 serving

► **Variations:** Add ⅛ teaspoon ground cinnamon, ½ teaspoon instant decaffeinated coffee powder, ⅛ teaspoon vanilla extract, or ⅛ teaspoon coconut extract.

► **Cooking tip:** In the summer, if your blender can crush ice, you can make frozen hot cocoa: let hot cocoa cool, then put in blender with one ice cube and blend until frothy.

SERVING GUIDELINES

► **FOR EVERYONE WHO'S HAD BARIATRIC SURGERY:**
   Week 1: Liquid diet.
   Weeks 2+: Serve as is.

► **FOR OTHERS:**
   Serve as is.

Calories: 98, **Protein:** 9 g, **Fat:** 1 g, **Carbohydrates:** 16 g, **Cholesterol:** 5 mg, **Fiber:** 2 g, **Sodium:** 129 mg

Savory & Sweet Sauces

Versatile entrée and dessert sauces layer on taste and texture

WAIT A MINUTE. Can you really eat sauces? Aren't you trying to lose weight? The answer is yes to both. All these sauce recipes are low in calories and carbs and have no added sugars. What they do have is lots of flavor.

Sauces are very important for two reasons: First, during your early postoperative period, you'll need some kind of liquid base to make a smooth puree, and these sauces work perfectly and taste amazing. Second, if you try to lose weight by eating nothing but dry broiled and baked food for the rest of your life, you'll be miserable and probably cheat or just give up. With these delicious sauces, you can eat right and enjoy every mouthful.

In this section you'll find both savory and sweet sauces. A savory sauce can be a creamy sauce with a horseradish punch or a mixture of chopped vegetables with wine and broth; a quick, light tomato sauce; a spicy salsa; or a tangy mixture of fresh plums, tomato paste, and spices. Our sweet sauces include a surprisingly luscious chocolate sauce, but you'll also discover fresh fruit sauces that are versatile enough to top one of our low-fat desserts, perk up a plain piece of chicken or fish, or stir into yogurt (plain, fat-free yogurt, of course).

So, sauce it up and enjoy your meals even more. With our sauces there's no reason not to.

Note: The nutritional analyses are based on a two-tablespoon serving.

Asian Dipping Sauce

This is our version of the classic sauce that's often served with dumplings and other Chinese appetizers.

¾ cup light soy sauce

¼ cup rice vinegar

2 teaspoons red pepper flakes, or to taste

1 teaspoon sesame oil

1 or 2 packets artificial sweetener
   (or to taste)

1. In a small bowl, combine all ingredients and mix well.
2. Cover and let stand for 10 to 20 minutes to let flavors blend before serving.

Makes approximately 1 cup

➤ **Hint:** This sauce can be refrigerated for up to 1 week. It makes a great liquid base for purees.

➤ **Serving suggestions:** Try it with our Asian Turkey-Filled Cabbage Dumplings (page 80) or Singapore Shrimp Dumplings (page 155). It's also tasty with simple broiled chicken or fish.

Calories: 15, **Protein:** 1 g, **Fat:** 0 g, **Carbohydrates:** 2 g, **Cholesterol:** 0 mg, **Fiber:** 0 g, **Sodium:** 407 mg

Caesar Sauce

This is a low-fat version of the classic Caesar dressing. But why just stop at salads? It's a tasty addition to lots of dishes.

¼ cup Dijon mustard
¼ cup grated Parmesan cheese
4 garlic cloves, minced
2 tablespoons anchovy paste
2 tablespoons Worcestershire sauce
¼ cup balsamic vinegar
¼ cup plain, fat-free yogurt

1. Combine all ingredients in a blender or food processor and puree until smooth.

Makes approximately 1 cup

➤ **Hint:** This sauce makes a great liquid base for purees.
➤ **Serving suggestions:** This sauce is extremely versatile—you can try it on fish or chicken, use as a salad dressing, toss with cooked green vegetables (serve hot or cold), and even add some prepared horseradish and serve with cold beef or veal.

Calories: 25, **Protein:** 1 g, **Fat:** 1 g, **Carbohydrates:** 3 g, **Cholesterol:** 9 mg, **Fiber:** 0 g, **Sodium:** 230 mg

Garlic Sauce

This pungent sauce is a delicious way to enhance the flavor of simple roasted, broiled, or poached foods. You can serve it hot or cold.

½ cup plain, fat-free yogurt
4 garlic cloves, finely minced
1 tablespoon fresh lemon juice
½ cup low-sodium chicken broth

1. Pour yogurt into a fine-mesh strainer over a small bowl and let stand for 15 minutes. Discard any liquid that has drained from yogurt.
2. In a small bowl, crush garlic until it forms a paste, then stir in lemon juice.
3. Add drained yogurt to garlic mixture and stir well.
4. In a small saucepan, bring chicken broth to a simmer, stir in yogurt-garlic mixture, and simmer for 1 minute more, stirring constantly.

Makes approximately 1 cup
➤ **Hint:** This sauce makes a great liquid base for purees.
➤ **Serving suggestions:** A perfect topping for beef, lamb, chicken, turkey loaf—even poached fish.

Calories: 7, **Protein:** 1 g, **Fat:** 0 g, **Carbohydrates:** 1 g, **Cholesterol:** 0 mg, **Fiber:** 0 g, **Sodium:** 29 mg

Spicy-Creamy Citrus Sauce

This creamy sauce is a fusion of Asian and Cuban flavors—cool, yet hot.

½ cup fat-free sour cream
2 tablespoons low-sodium soy sauce
2 tablespoons fresh lime juice
2 tablespoons fresh orange juice
Brown-sugar artificial sweetener
   (½ teaspoon equivalent)
½ teaspoon Asian chili paste with garlic
1 tablespoon finely grated fresh ginger
¼ cup chopped fresh basil

1. In a small bowl, combine all ingredients and mix well. If not using right away, refrigerate. Sauce can be refrigerated in a tightly sealed container up to 1 week.
2. Bring sauce to room temperature when ready to serve.

Makes approximately 1 cup

➤ **Hint:** This sauce makes a great liquid base for purees.
➤ **Serving suggestions:** This sauce tastes excellent on baked or broiled shrimp, salmon, swordfish, or tuna. You can also use it as a dipping sauce for shrimp cocktail.

Calories: 14, **Protein:** 1 g, **Fat:** 0 g, **Carbohydrates:** 2 g, **Cholesterol:** 1 mg, **Fiber:** 0 g, **Sodium:** 76 mg

Citrus-Horseradish Sauce

This creamy topping gets its heat from horseradish and its cool freshness from citrus. It's a quick uncooked sauce that can liven up lots of dishes.

½ cup fat-free sour cream
½ cup low-fat mayonnaise
1 teaspoon grated lemon zest
1 tablespoon fresh lemon juice
1 teaspoon grated lime zest
1 tablespoon fresh lime juice
2 teaspoons capers, drained
2 teaspoons prepared white horseradish
½ cup fresh basil leaves, finely chopped

1. Combine all ingredients in a small bowl and whisk until smooth.

Makes approximately 1 cup

► **Hint:** This sauce makes a great liquid base for purees.
► **Serving suggestions:** This is delicious as a sauce for fish, chicken, pork, or beef. You can also use it as a base for tuna, egg, or salmon salad, and it works well as a salad dressing or tossed with cold or hot cooked vegetables.

Calories: 36, **Protein:** 1 g, **Fat:** 3 g, **Carbohydrates:** 2 g, **Cholesterol:** 4 mg, **Fiber:** 0 g, **Sodium:** 84 mg

Creamy Basil-Seafood Sauce

This sauce packs a powerful punch, so you just need to use a little bit. It makes a terrific glaze as well as a sauce for broiled or baked fish.

½ cup fat-free sour cream
½ cup low-fat mayonnaise
2 tablespoons prepared horseradish
¼ cup chopped fresh basil
2 teaspoons light soy sauce
2 tablespoons minced onion
1 teaspoon minced fresh ginger
1 tablespoon anchovy paste

1. Combine all ingredients in a medium bowl and mix well.

Makes approximately 1 cup

► **Hint:** This sauce makes a great liquid base for purees.
► **Serving suggestions:** This sauce gives you a tangy way to perk up poached or broiled fish. You can also mix it into tuna or salmon salad instead of mayonnaise or use it as a dip for vegetables or cold steamed shrimp.

Calories: 39, **Protein:** 1 g, **Fat:** 3 g, **Carbohydrates:** 3 g, **Cholesterol:** 7 mg, **Fiber:** 0 g, **Sodium:** 166 mg

Shallot-Horseradish Sauce

Creamy with a bit of a kick, this lovely pale-pink sauce dresses up even the simplest of entrées.

Canola cooking spray
¼ cup minced shallots
1½ teaspoons minced garlic
¼ cup white wine
1 tablespoon condensed chicken broth
¾ cup plain, fat-free yogurt
1 teaspoon sweet paprika
1 tablespoon prepared horseradish

1. Coat a small nonstick saucepan with cooking spray and sauté shallots and garlic over medium-high heat until soft but not browned.
2. Add white wine and condensed chicken broth, lower heat, and bring to a slow simmer.
3. Add yogurt, paprika, and horseradish and cook, barely simmering, for 5 minutes, or until slightly reduced.

Makes approximately 1 cup

➤ **Hint:** This sauce makes a great liquid base for purees.
➤ **Serving suggestions:** This makes a tangy addition to broiled or sautéed chicken, turkey, or pork. You can also serve cold with beef or lamb.

Calories: 16, **Protein:** 1 g, **Fat:** 0 g, **Carbohydrates:** 2 g, **Cholesterol:** 0 mg, **Fiber:** 0 g, **Sodium:** 79 mg

Simple Horseradish Sauce

It couldn't be easier—no cutting, no chopping, no cooking—just a piquant, bold taste that adds a kick to even the most basic dishes.

1 cup fat-free sour cream

3 tablespoons concentrated chicken broth

2 teaspoons sweet paprika

2 tablespoons prepared horseradish

1. In a small bowl, combine all ingredients and mix well. If not using right away, refrigerate. Sauce can be refrigerated in a tightly sealed container up to 1 week.

2. Bring sauce to room temperature when ready to serve.

Makes approximately 1 cup

➤ **Hint:** This sauce makes a great liquid base for purees.

➤ **Serving suggestions:** This sauce is great on broiled beef or chicken, sautéed chicken or turkey cutlets, and can really sauce up a turkey burger.

Calories: 24, **Protein:** 1 g, **Fat:** 1 g, **Carbohydrates:** 4 g, **Cholesterol:** 54 mg, **Fiber:** 0 g, **Sodium:** 202 mg

Creamy Wasabi Sauce

Adding Asian ingredients to a creamy base makes this unusual sauce delicious as well as very versatile.

½ cup fat-free sour cream
½ cup low-fat mayonnaise
1 tablespoon light soy sauce
1 packet artificial sweetener
   (Splenda or Truvia)
2 teaspoons wasabi paste

1. Mix all ingredients together in a small bowl until well blended.

Makes approximately 1 cup
- ► **Hint:** This sauce makes a great liquid base for purees.
- ► **Serving suggestions:** Use this sauce to add just a hint of heat to fish and shrimp, try it as a dip with raw vegetables, or mix it into tuna, chicken, or salmon salad instead of plain mayonnaise.

Calories: 37, **Protein:** 1 g, **Fat:** 3 g, **Carbohydrates:** 3 g, **Cholesterol:** 4 mg, **Fiber:** 0 g, **Sodium:** 110 mg

Quick Tomato Sauce

For years I've made my own slow-cooked tomato sauce with fresh plum tomatoes. But when fresh tomatoes are not in season, or when I just don't have the time, I make this light, simple version.

Olive oil cooking spray
1 garlic clove, minced
1 (14.5-ounce) can diced tomatoes
1 packet artificial sweetener
  (Splenda or Truvia)
2 tablespoons chopped fresh basil leaves

1. In a medium nonstick saucepan, heat cooking spray over medium heat, add garlic, and sauté until slightly browned.
2. Add tomatoes, sweetener, and basil, lower heat, and simmer for 5 to 7 minutes.

Makes approximately 1 cup

➤ **Hint:** This sauce makes a great liquid base for purees.
➤ **Serving suggestions:** This topping gives a light, Italian accent to fish, chicken, meatloaf, turkey loaf, or meatballs. You can also spoon it on sautéed or broiled sliced steak.

Calories: 8.79, **Protein:** 0.44 g, **Fat:** 0 g, **Carbohydrates:** 1.82 g, **Cholesterol:** 0 mg, **Fiber:** 0.44 g, **Sodium:** 40.06 mg

Sauce Piperade

This is similar to our Sauce Basquaise but without the wine and beef broth, just lots of lovely fresh vegetables and garlic.

Olive oil cooking spray
¼ cup chopped onion
1 garlic clove, chopped
¼ cup seeded and diced green bell pepper
¼ cup seeded and diced red bell pepper
¼ pound white mushrooms, sliced
¼ cup seeded and chopped plum tomatoes
Salt and pepper to taste

1. Coat a medium nonstick lidded skillet with cooking spray. Over a medium-high heat, sauté onion and garlic until lightly browned.
2. Lower heat to medium, add bell peppers and mushrooms to pan, and cook, covered, for 3 to 5 minutes, or until soft.
3. Add tomatoes and cook, stirring occasionally, for 2 minutes or until tomatoes have softened and sauce has thickened. Add salt and pepper to taste.

Makes approximately 1 cup

➤ **Hint:** This sauce makes a great liquid base for purees.
➤ **Serving suggestions:** Try stirring this sauce into scrambled eggs or folding into an omelet. It's also delicious with any kind of fish or seafood and terrific for topping a chicken or turkey cutlet.

Calories: 5, **Protein:** 0 g, **Fat:** 0 g, **Carbohydrates:** 1 g, **Cholesterol:** 0 mg, **Fiber:** 0 g, **Sodium:** 1 mg

Sauce Basquaise

This started out as a traditional Basque sauce—peppers, tomatoes, and onions—then we added lots of other good stuff.

Olive oil cooking spray
¼ cup chopped onion
1 garlic clove, chopped
¼ cup seeded and diced green bell pepper
¼ cup seeded and diced red bell pepper
¼ pound white mushrooms, sliced
¼ cup red wine
¼ cup seeded and chopped plum tomatoes
1½ teaspoons concentrated beef broth
Salt and pepper to taste

1. Coat a medium nonstick lidded skillet with cooking spray and sauté onion and garlic over a medium-high heat until lightly browned.
2. Lower heat to medium, add bell peppers and mushrooms to pan, and cook, covered, for 3 to 5 minutes, or until soft.
3. Add wine, tomatoes, and beef broth concentrate and cook, stirring occasionally, for 3 minutes, or until sauce has thickened and reduced by half. Add salt and pepper to taste.

Makes approximately 1 cup
- **Hint:** This sauce makes a great liquid base for purees.
- **Serving suggestions:** This sauce is excellent with beef (steak, London broil, meatloaf, burgers, or meatballs) and also works well with lamb or veal.

Calories: 11, **Protein:** 0 g, **Fat:** 0 g, **Carbohydrates:** 1 g, **Cholesterol:** 0 mg, **Fiber:** 0 g, **Sodium:** 45 mg

Yogurt-Mint Sauce

This sauce represents a classic Greek blend of flavors—cool and minty, with the tanginess of lemon and yogurt.

¾ cup plain, fat-free yogurt
1 small garlic clove, quartered
1 teaspoon ground cumin
½ teaspoon lemon zest
1 tablespoon fresh lemon juice
½ cup mint leaves
2 teaspoons chicken broth concentrate

1. Place all ingredients in a food processor and puree until smooth.

Makes approximately 1 cup

➤ **Hint:** This sauce makes a great liquid base for purees.
➤ **Serving suggestions:** This Mediterranean way to spark up lamb and swordfish also makes a good salad dressing. Try mixing it with cooked vegetables or using it as a dip for crudités.

Calories: 15, **Protein:** 1 g, **Fat:** 0 g, **Carbohydrates:** 3 g, **Cholesterol:** 0 mg, **Fiber:** 1 g, **Sodium:** 52 mg

Tikka Yogurt Sauce

This classic Indian sauce blends a complex mix of spices into a taste bud–tingling experience.

Canola cooking spray
1 tablespoon minced garlic
¾ cup plain low-fat yogurt
¼ cup low-sodium chicken broth
½ small red chile, seeded and minced
½ teaspoon ground cumin
½ teaspoon ground coriander
½ teaspoon ground turmeric
½ teaspoon garam masala
2 tablespoons fresh lime juice
Salt and pepper to taste

1. Coat a small saucepan with cooking spray and sauté garlic until soft.
2. Add all other ingredients and cook over low heat for 3 minutes.

Makes approximately 1 cup
➤ **Hint:** This sauce makes a great liquid base for purees.
➤ **Serving suggestions:** This sauce gives an Indian accent to fish and chicken dishes. It also makes a great salad dressing, or can be mixed with cooked vegetables, served hot or cold.

Calories: 11, **Protein:** 1 g, **Fat:** 0 g, **Carbohydrates:** 2 g, **Cholesterol:** 0 mg, **Fiber:** 0 g, **Sodium:** 23 mg

Sweet-and-Sour Sauce

If you have or had a grandma from one of the Middle European countries or Russia, you probably remember her savory sweet-and-sour recipes. With that taste memory as a guideline, we created this lighter, more citrusy version.

Cooking spray
¼ cup minced onion
1½ teaspoons minced fresh ginger
1½ teaspoons tomato paste
1 (8-ounce) can no-salt-added
   tomato sauce
2 tablespoons fresh orange juice
1½ teaspoons red wine vinegar
1 packet artificial sweetener
   (Splenda or Truvia)

1. In a large nonstick skillet, heat cooking spray until hot but not smoking.
2. Sauté onion until just soft but not browned. Add ginger and stir for 30 seconds. Add all other ingredients and simmer for 5 minutes.

Makes approximately 1 cup
- ➤ **Hint:** This sauce makes a great liquid base for purees.
- ➤ **Serving suggestions:** You can use this as the sauce for our Sweet-and-Sour Stuffed Cabbage (page 78) or try it as a topping on broiled halibut or swordfish. It's delicious mixed with beef or turkey meatballs, and it also tastes great on poached or broiled chicken.

Calories: 8, **Protein:** 0 g, **Fat:** 0 g, **Carbohydrates:** 2 g, **Cholesterol:** 0 mg, **Fiber:** 0 g, **Sodium:** 7 mg

Fresh Plum Sauce

This is one of those extremely versatile recipes that I just adore. It adds another dimension of flavor to a wide variety of foods—from Asian recipes to Indian curries, and even to good old American comfort food.

Canola cooking spray
½ cup chopped onion
3 large red or purple plums, pitted
   and chopped
1 garlic clove, minced
1 tablespoon tomato paste
½ small jalapeño pepper, seeded and
   minced
1 tablespoon balsamic vinegar
1 tablespoon light soy sauce
Brown-sugar artificial sweetener
   (1 teaspoon equivalent)

1. Coat a nonstick saucepan with cooking spray, heat over medium-high, and sauté onion until just translucent.
2. Add all other ingredients, lower heat, and cook over low heat for 10 minutes, or until thick.
3. Let cool slightly, pour into a food processor, and blend until smooth.

Makes approximately 1 cup
► **Hint:** This sauce makes a great liquid base for purees.
► **Serving suggestions:** This sauce adds a tangy note to pork, poultry, and shrimp. You can also use it as a cooking glaze or a dipping sauce. I often use it in place of hoisin sauce. Thin it out with a little more soy and vinegar and use it as a marinade. Serve it as a condiment with Indian or Pakistani curries. It also makes a great substitute for ketchup (much lower in sugar) on meatloaf, or mixed into your meatloaf recipe (2 tablespoons) before cooking.

Calories: 12, **Protein:** 0 g, **Fat:** 0 g, **Carbohydrates:** 3 g, **Cholesterol:** 0 mg, **Fiber:** 0 g, **Sodium:** 49 mg

Mango Salsa

I love fruit sauces, especially savory salsas, like this one, that contrast the sweetness of fresh tropical fruit with the heat of chili. Of course, if you really like it hot, increase the chili powder or add a whole minced hot pepper.

¼ cup low-sodium chicken broth
¾ cup diced fresh ripe mango
⅓ cup thinly sliced red onion
1 tablespoon balsamic vinegar
½ packet artificial sweetener
   (Splenda or Truvia)
1 teaspoon chili powder

1 In a small saucepan, bring chicken broth to a slow boil.
2. Add all other ingredients and cook for about 10 minutes, or until thick.
3. Puree for a smooth sauce, or serve chunky.

Makes approximately 1 cup

➤ **Hint:** This sauce makes a great liquid base for purees. Can be refrigerated, tightly sealed, for up to 2 weeks.

➤ **Serving suggestions:** Use this sauce to really zing up regular or smoked pork chops, chicken, or stronger-flavored fish, such as fresh salmon, tuna, swordfish, or shrimp. It also makes a delicious dip.

Calories: 8, **Protein:** 0 g, **Fat:** 0 g, **Carbohydrates:** 2 g, **Cholesterol:** 0 mg, **Fiber:** 0 g, **Sodium:** 27 mg

Papaya Salsa

Combining the mellow sweetness of papaya with the hot kick of chili powder is a very tropical tradition.

¼ cup low-sodium chicken broth
¾ cup diced fresh, very ripe papaya
⅓ cup thinly sliced red onion
1 tablespoon balsamic vinegar
½ packet artificial sweetener
   (Splenda or Truvia)
1 teaspoon chili powder

1. In a small saucepan, bring chicken broth to a slow boil.
2. Add all other ingredients and cook about 10 minutes until thick.
3. Puree for a smooth sauce or serve chunky.

Makes approximately 1 cup
- **Hint:** This sauce makes a great liquid base for purees.
- **Serving suggestions:** This sauce adds some spark to regular or smoked pork chops, chicken, or stronger-flavored fish, such as fresh salmon, tuna, swordfish, or shrimp. It also makes a tasty dip.

Calories: 5, **Protein:** 0 g, **Fat:** 0 g, **Carbohydrates:** 1 g, **Cholesterol:** 0 mg, **Fiber:** 0 g, **Sodium:** 27 mg

Pineapple Salsa

There's nothing better than the sweet juiciness of a fresh pineapple, except maybe this fresh pineapple salsa.

1 cup chopped fresh pineapple
3 tablespoons fresh orange juice
1½ teaspoons red-wine vinegar
1 teaspoon red chili paste
1 teaspoon minced garlic
¼ teaspoon sesame oil
Brown-sugar artificial sweetener
   (1 teaspoon equivalent)

1. Combine all ingredients in a food processor and pulse until coarsely blended.

Makes approximately 1 cup

➤ **Hint:** This sauce makes a great liquid base for purees.
➤ **Serving suggestions:** This is a classic salsa that really livens up meat, poultry, shrimp, or fish. You can also use it as a dip.

Calories: 7, **Protein:** 0 g, **Fat:** 0 g, **Carbohydrates:** 2 g, **Cholesterol:** 0 mg, **Fiber:** 0 g, **Sodium:** 2 mg

Chocolate Sauce

We couldn't believe it when we created this thick, rich-tasting sauce that has virtually no fat. It's real chocolate sauce, no kidding.

1 cup evaporated skim milk
½ cup unsweetened cocoa powder
6 packets artificial sweetener
   (Splenda or Truvia)

1. In a small saucepan, bring evaporated milk to a simmer.
2. Pour ¼ cup of heated milk into a small bowl and stir in cocoa powder until it forms a smooth paste.
3. Simmer rest of milk for 2 to 3 minutes to reduce and thicken slightly.
4. Add cocoa paste and sweetener to milk in saucepan and stir over low heat until smooth.
5. Chill, covered, in refrigerator for at least 1 hour (if too thick, stir in a little more evaporated milk until it reaches desired consistency).
6. Can be served hot, like hot fudge sauce, or at room temperature.

Makes approximately 1 cup

► **Serving suggestions:** This luscious topping tastes fantastic on the Flan (page 177). You can also try pouring it over water-packed canned or poached fruit or using it as a topping on fat-free, sugar-free ice cream or frozen yogurt.

Calories: 19, **Protein:** 2 g, **Fat:** 0 g, **Carbohydrates:** 4 g, **Cholesterol:** 0 mg, **Fiber:** 1 g, **Sodium:** 21 mg

Raspberry Sauce

This is a bright, tangy sauce that, thanks to the availability of fresh-frozen raspberries, tastes like summer all year long.

1 cup fresh-frozen raspberries
6 packets artificial sweetener
   (Splenda or Truvia)
½ cup water
1 tablespoon fresh lemon juice

1. In a saucepan, mix raspberries, sweetener, water, and lemon juice and bring to a boil, then lower heat and simmer for 10 minutes.
2. Remove from heat; let cool, then strain through a fine sieve into a bowl, pressing down to catch all liquids. Discard seeds and solids.
3. Cover and chill in refrigerator for 30 minutes.

Makes approximately 1 cup

➤ **Serving suggestions:** This classic topping tastes amazing on the Flan (page 177), Basic Cheesecake (page 174), and Lemon Soufflé (page 178) recipes. Try pouring it over water-packed canned or poached fruit and fat-free, sugar-free ice cream or frozen yogurt. You can even mix it into plain, fat-free yogurt.

Calories: 4, **Protein:** 0 g, **Fat:** 0 g, **Carbohydrates:** 1 g, **Cholesterol:** 0 mg, **Fiber:** 1 g, **Sodium:** 0 mg

Strawberry Sauce

While you can probably make this sauce with frozen strawberries, I prefer to wait for really ripe, fresh berries.

1 cup hulled and sliced fresh strawberries
½ cup water
6 packets artificial sweetener
   (Splenda or Truvia)
½ teaspoon balsamic vinegar

1. In a small saucepan, combine sauce ingredients and bring to a boil. Lower heat and simmer for 10 minutes, stirring occasionally, until strawberries are soft and sauce is slightly thickened.
2. Pour into a container cover, and chill for at least 4 hours.

Makes approximately 1 cup

➤ **Serving suggestions:** This classic topping tastes great on the Flan (page 177), Basic Cheesecake (page 174), Lemon Soufflé (page 178), and Strawberry Ricotta Whip (page 176) recipes. You can also try pouring it over water-packed canned or poached fruit and as a topping on fat-free, sugar-free ice cream or frozen yogurt. You can even mix it into plain, fat-free yogurt.

Calories: 7, **Protein:** 0 g, **Fat:** 0 g, **Carbohydrates:** 2 g, **Cholesterol:** 0 mg, **Fiber:** 1 g, **Sodium:** 5 mg

Papaya Sauce

Here's a perfect way to add a light taste of the Tropics to low-fat, low-carb desserts. But don't stop at desserts; this is a very versatile sauce for main dishes, too.

½ large very ripe papaya (about 1 cup)
¼ teaspoon vanilla extract
1 tablespoon fresh lime juice
Artificial sweetener (Splenda or Truvia)
   to taste (optional)

1. Peel and seed papaya and scoop flesh into a food processor or blender.
2. Add vanilla and lime juice and puree until very smooth (if sauce is not sweet enough, add artificial sweetener to taste).

Makes approximately 1 cup

➤ **Serving suggestions:** This works wonderfully as either a savory meal sauce or a dessert sauce. Try it with poultry, pork, or shrimp, or use as a topping for the luscious Flan recipe (page 177). Pour over fat-free, sugar-free ice cream or frozen yogurt, or mix into plain, fat-free yogurt.

Calories: 4, **Protein:** 0 g, **Fat:** 0 g, **Carbohydrates:** 1 g, **Cholesterol:** 0 mg, **Fiber:** 0 g, **Sodium:** 0 mg

Acknowledgments

WHILE WE HAVE too many supportive friends and family members to list individually, there are a few who we'd like to especially acknowledge. Thank you to Bob Levine, my adoring and adorable husband of many years, and our primary guinea pig (who, by the way, lost a lot of weight on our eating program). Thank you to Michael Saray, Michele's fabulous husband, partner, and best friend, for his unwavering support and pride in her newest accomplishment. To Elyse Schapira, Michele's sister, for her early advice and assistance. A warm thanks to Meredith Urban-Skuro, for not only helping me to start a new way of life both physically and emotionally, but for all her enthusiasm and involvement in this book. Thank you to my surgeon, Dr. Inabnet, who contributed to the first edition of this book. Thank you to Dr. William Suozzi, the primary care physician for Bob and me, as well as for Michele and Michael, who had the compassion to suggest and discuss the possibility of weight-reduction surgery for me. Thank you to Deirdre Mullane, without whom we might never have found our way to our first publisher. And, thank you so much to Matthew Lore, the incredible publisher of the first edition, who knew from the very beginning what we were talking about and just how to help us accomplish it. And we can't forget Peter Jacoby, Matthew's assistant, for all his invaluable assistance. Thank you to Suzanne McCloskey, our first editor, for all her patience and very smart suggestions. And, finally, our newest thank you to Claire Schulz and her team at Da Capo Lifelong Books and Hachette Book Group, who convinced me that it was time to update the cookbook and add new recipes.

Thank you all so much.

Index

About the Authors

PATT LEVINE is a professional writer who has been a serious cook for many years. In addition to her long career in advertising as an executive-level copywriter for both retail stores and advertising agencies, she has had recipes published in *Gourmet* magazine. After battling weight problems since her early thirties, she decided to have weight reduction surgery in April 2003. Realizing that she would have to drastically change her way of cooking and eating after surgery, she developed a high-protein, low-fat food program that includes everything from soup to dessert. Working with her coauthor, Michele Bontempo, Patt has combined her two areas of expertise in this cookbook to help other people who have had, or are thinking of having, weight-reduction surgery to achieve their weight-loss goals while enjoying delicious food. Patt graduated from the Fashion Institute of Technology in New York City with a degree in communications. In addition to writing, she designs most of her own clothes, has been a professional singer, and has taught advertising copywriting at two New York colleges. Longtime New Yorkers, Patt, her husband, Bob, and their two cats, Jazz and Quincy, now live in rural Connecticut.

MICHELE BONTEMPO is an art director and graphic designer who has worked in both the fashion and home furnishing fields. Her career has included positions in some of New York's top department stores as well as a number of advertising, design, and catalog agencies. She and her business partner, Richard Oreiro, also ran their own advertising catalog and design agency for ten years. Known for her innate sense of "what looks right," Michele has also been involved in a number of corporate identification and interior design projects. Michele was born in London, England, and grew up in the Bronx, New York. She has also lived in Italy and Canada. She and her husband, Michael, live in New York City.